By His Stripes...

Healed of MS

By His Stripes...

Healed of MS

PATTI BESYK

with

Cliff Dudley

New Leaf 🕊 Press

P.O. BOX 311, GREEN FOREST, AR 72638

FIRST EDITION
1986

Editor: Dale Dawson

Typesetting by SPACE
Berryville, Arkansas 72616

Library of Congress Catalog Card Number: 86-061068
International Standard Book Number:0-89221-141-5

Printed in the United States of America

Cover Photo: Cover Studio Photography
Johnstown, PA

TABLE OF CONTENTS

DEDICATION

To my husband Frank: without his loving patience and quiet strength throughout my terrible illness, this story might have had a different and unhappy ending.

To my parents: they bore the brunt of unimaginable sorrow and pain as they had to watch their only daughter slip from their grasp as they did all they humanly could to help. They raised my son for almost five years and showed me nothing but love and patience.

To my son Brett: whose baby years were a confusing maze of baby sitters, living at two homes and having a mother who could only sit by and watch him grow up; yet through it all he still would say, "Mommy I love you."

FOREWORD

When a person has been called to the healing ministry of the Lord Jesus Christ by the Lord Jesus Himself, and gently, but very firmly taught to leave the results of that ministry up the the Lord, I can easily imagine that that person could have a deep, although unaware, desire to have that ministry vindicated by a reliable authority, under the guidance of the Holy Spirit, in his own lifetime.

If this were so, then that reliable authority should be someone quite close to that person.

This is what happened in this life story of the healing of Patti Besyk of MS by the Lord Jesus, for this one called to the healing ministry was her pastor and friend during most of Patti's growing up years, and could not have chosen a better example to be this reliable authority.

As my Lord Jesus gives me this foreword, I have an ever deeper realization that all of the marvelous events concerning Patti's healing have been under the direct guidance of the Holy Spirit. I also realize afresh that the writing of her life story has brought about an additional vindication of the glorious healing gospel of the Lord Jesus Christ.

As you read this interesting story of Patti's life I trust that you will feel like praying with me what King David prayed in I Chronicles 29:11,

"Thine, O Lord, is the greatness, and the power, and the glory, and the victory, and the majesty: for all that is in the heaven and the earth is thine: thine is the kingdom, O Lord, and thou art exalted as head above all."

Amen!

George A. Clark
Waynesboro, PA

7

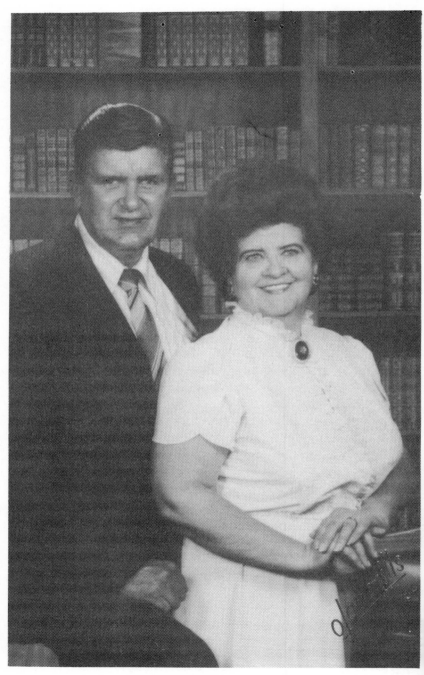

Patti's Mom and Dad
Betty and Karl

1

Coal Miner's Daughter

Life is different in the rolling hills and rugged mountains of Pennsylvania. If you are from a large city like New York or Chicago, the contrast may seem somewhat hayseed by comparison. It's different because there are values and a closeness, or kinship, that are often lost or muffled in the busyness of more metropolitan lifestyles. Things change, even in small communities, but those deeper things (like values) remain, for the most part, constant. Maybe that's the way God intended it.

The people of rural Pennsylvania are proud people, men and women of character and compassion, qualities passed down (like heirlooms) from generation to generation. Youthful rebellion is nothing new. It's been happening since the offspring of Adam and Eve. It's just more publicized today. But in the Bible it says if you bring up your kids showing them how they should live their lives that, after their youthful rebellions, they'll come back to those values. That's the way things are in rural Pennsylvania, a state blessed with natural beauty, and people who know there's an Almighty God, and do the best they can do to live by His rules, whether they go to church or not! That's just the way it is, and you don't argue with their faith. If you're smart, you learn from it!

One who is prone to the comforts and conveniences of a more metropolitan lifestyle might not survive one four-season cycle in rural Pennsylvania. The seasons have a beauty and brutality which could quickly destroy a weakling. But this combination of beauty and brutality has honed and polished the hidden qualities which lie dormant for a lifetime in most of us. When your house sets one or two-hundred feet back off a one or two-lane dirt or gravel road and a fierce blizzard buries you in an instant winter wonderland, you don't call a plowing service -- you bundle up real good, get out your shovel, and start digging! Not only do you dig a path from your car or truck to the gravel road, but you keep digging, down the road, until you either meet up with a county snow plow or you give up!

If there's no reason to "dig out," you don't bother. City folks might panic in the same situation, but country folks adapt. City folks depend on the local supermarket for their next meal; country folks rely on themselves, and what God's given them in the good seasons to see them through the rough ones. When you're "snowed in," you go to the pantry or fruit cellar and build a meal from your canned goods, not goods in "cans", but what you have canned (a nearly lost art in the city) from past seasons. And when the pantry or fruit cellar shelves are nearing bare, you make do with what you have, and when the shelves are completely bare, you pray, and somehow you survive. That's how it is sometimes and you accept it, because that's how you were brought up, to teach us a very uncomplicated form of faith, trust and acceptance.

Jerome, Boswell, Hollsopple, Thomas Mill, Davidsville, even Tire Hill. These names mean nothing to most people, nor should they. But these strange-sounding names mean the world to me, Patti Besyk, because they are, literally, my "world". If you check an atlas, you will find these tiny specks just south of

Johnstown. They are like any other small clusters of townspeople anywhere else in the United States. To most folks they are "the boon-docks", "hicksville", but to me they are important because that is where the Lord has placed me. Not unlike Jesus in His earthly walk, I have been limited to a very small geographical circle on a very large globe, but it is the acreage God has given me, and I am content with it.

My growing-up years were no different than a thousand (or million) others in our great land. I was raised in rural America by loving parents who did the best they knew how in parenting me. In those growing-up years, my name was Patti Coughenour. My mother is a short, strong and loving German. My dad, a tall, proud "German-Swede". Because of his last name, he was always called "Coke" by his closer friends, number one being his beloved wife. As a couple, they looked like Mutt and Jeff, but anybody who knows them knows they have never been "two", but "one" in the spirit of their marriage.

Dad is a deeply caring husband, father and friend, but is not a man of open emotion or affection. On a deeper level, these are things you accept in a person, and Dad has always been a good person. I have never doubted that. As a transplanted German-Swede in the hills of Pennsylvania, Dad probably never doubted his marriage vows: you get married; you take care of your wife and are faithful to her; you produce a family; you raise them and you provide for them. In a traditional upbringing, that's the way it is, with no gray areas in thinking! I believe that's the way God meant it to be.

There is no doubt that my parents had their disagreements, debates, differences and downright arguments, but for the most part, the home-front was stable in my upbringing. I did have a problem in dealing with being the only girl out of four children. Harold, Ron and Terry were the boys. I (in my own mind) was the oddball. In trying to compensate for being a female in this setting, I developed into quite a "tomboy" during my school years. Perhaps my early motivations were unfounded, but they probably had some foundation. Being raised in a very (traditionally) male supremacy environment, it would have been easy for me to begin to compete at a very early age. In current terms, it was a "no fault" situation: my parents were raising all of their children with values which had been instilled in them, yet I always felt like I must compete for either attention or acceptance. Even when no scars are intended, they often result.

Recess was the loneliest, most frustrating time in those early school years for me. When the girls were playing little girl games (hopscotch or whatever), I would often sit on the school steps alone, sometimes crying, because I didn't fit in. I was supposed to be playing little girl games, but I yearned to be playing baseball or football with the boys. I was even competing with my brothers in the school yard. Did I want to prove myself or be accepted by my brothers, my father? Only God knows. Competition between children in any family is sometimes fierce (parents seldom understand or acknowledge this), but in a family with three boys and just one girl, it is more difficult than any parent can realize. I learned the spirit of competition at a very early age. That "spirit" caused me many scars in later years, some real, some imagined, and some self-inflicted. By the way, I did finally learn to play hopscotch.

It's not that my parents weren't proud of me and didn't encourage me to grow up as a girl. Maybe they were just in two different emotional arenas. On the one hand, I always felt I had to compete with my three brothers for acceptance, while, on the other hand, Dad and Mom may have looked upon me as the one daughter out of four children, as maybe a special gift of God. I never saw it that way in those growing-up years.

Dad is, and has always been, an even-tempered man. But when his fur got ruffled, he would react, whether on the job, or at home. And it didn't matter if his fur was ruffled by his spouse or one of us kids. When he got ruffled, he got ruffled real good! He showed no partiality. Maybe Dad was even more stern with the boys than he would have been in a similar situation with me. I couldn't understand or accept that in those growing-up years. After all wasn't I one of the boys?

They farmed the limited land they had, but also had some chickens and a few cows. Obviously there were more chickens than cows. January in the hills of rural Pennsylvania is one of the colder, more rugged, months of the year. As it happened, the highest milk-producing Guernsey cow got loose. She didn't run away, but she ended up dying. Apparently this milk producer got out of her confines and curiosity or instinct led her to a full barrel of oats. Hunger and greed must have led her to eat the entire container of oats. As a result, this prize Guernsey bloated, and died. Dad didn't care so much that she had died as why! Since Harold was in charge of looking after the milk producer, Dad blamed him! Short and simple; no excuses.

The ground is frozen solid in Pennsylvania in January. Winter has set in and local residents conform to the supremacy of "mother nature's" hold on the landscape. Well, Dad didn't care what hold "mother nature" had on the hillsides of Pennsylvania. He judged that Harold was in charge of the livestock, and Harold has messed up in allowing the prize Guernsey to stray, so it was Harold's responsibility to dispose of the carcass! With Dad, everything was "black and white", no grey. Digging a grave for a human in Pennsylvania, in January, is one thing, but digging a hole for a cow carcass in frozen ground is something totally different, but Dad insisted on it, whether out of principle or stubbornness, so Harold dug the pit and buried the bloated carcass.

Yes, Dad had a temper. He had a financial loss with the dead cow, but with him it went deeper than that. With Harold, he was trying to instill deeper values. In short, Dad had placed Harold in charge, and the cow had eaten herself to death, so in Dad's mind, Harold was to blame! As a result, Harold ended up with hurt hands (and feelings) because he had to dig a very big hole in the frozen ground, in January, to bury the carcass of the Guernsey!! The cow probably could have been slaughtered, providing many meals through the sparse winter months, but Dad wouldn't entertain such a thought. In his mind, Harold had failed in his responsibility as the eldest male offspring, and slaughtering the cow would have let Harold off the hook too easily.

My brothers were constantly playing tricks on me. Maybe they were just "being boys", but they did test my little girl emotions. Most of my girl dolls ended up looking like Ken dolls long before Ken and Barbie were ever invented! For whatever reason, my brothers three got great joy out of sneaking into my room and cutting the hair off my dolls. My little girl baby dolls all ended up with crew cuts or stubble eventually. My Mom and Dad never found humor in these scalpings, and Dad would whip the boys, but the temporary stinging on their behinds never stopped them from continuing the pranks whenever they had opportunity or inclination. Let's face it, life was rough being the only girl.

Because I was the only girl, I helped my mother quite a bit with household chores. How I hated cleaning my dad's beat up aluminum lunch bucket. Scouring aluminum even when it's clean makes a mess, but a miner's lunch bucket is filthy after a shift underground. It would nearly gag me to have to clean it. Once when I was grumbling between swipes with the scouring pad, my Mom said, "Honey, as long as you're scrubbing that lunch bucket, your dad has a job." For some reason, that always stuck with me.

Coal miners, like their lunch pails, get filthy at their jobs hundreds and thousands of feet below the earth's surface. The crew may be integrated going into the mine, but they are all black-skinned when they emerge from the earth's belly. Because the first half-dozen years of my life were spent rather secluded on a small

Pennsylvania farm, I had never seen a black person. Even though I knew my daddy worked "in the mines," I had no idea what that meant, until this coal-dust-covered black man walked in the door one night. I was terrified and ran to my mother screaming and crying. Every exposed part of this stranger's body was literally coal black. It wasn't until the stranger spoke that I realized it was my daddy inside this stranger's body!

When your world is limited to the confines of a coal mining area, you don't know you're poor, because everybody is struggling, sometimes just to put the next meal on the table. Tennessee Ernie Ford had a song out in the mid-50's called "Sixteen Tons". Only a man who worked the mines in that era knows how true the lyrics were, "You load sixteen tons and what do you get? Another day older and deeper in debt. Saint Peter don't you call me 'cause I can't go. I owe my soul to the Company Store."

A lot of people over 30 are familiar with that song. Only those men who spent their lives below the ground filling their lungs with raw coal dust have lived the lyrics. In many Pennsylvania coal mining towns, not all, the mine company literally built and owned the town and its inhabitants! It was one of the truest forms of Socialism ever to operate within the free enterprise system. The mining company built rows of identical two-story wood-frame 2-bedroom, 4-room houses. Very simple; very basic. Even in the late 40's and early 50's, many were only equipped with outhouses, and all were heated, of course, with coal. The mining company would also build a "company store" in each of these communities of row houses, often called "patches". At these company stores you bought your groceries, your clothing and your kids store bought, Christmas gifts, all on credit. This was long before the days of Visa and MasterCard, but the end results were the same: people obligating their tomorrows to meet the needs of today! Whether it was for rent, food, coal or the other necessities, you literally owed your soul to the Company

Store, or at least, the coal mining company. The chances of ending up with any real folding money, after company deductions, at payday were slim at best.

Our family was more fortunate than many other miner families, for our modest farm home was not owned by the company. But still the six of us were a one-paycheck family, and life was a struggle. When you're a little kid, you don't think about where things come from; you just know they'll be there when they're supposed to be. If you're raised in a Christian upbringing, there is no doubt in your innocent little mind that Jesus will take care of blessing and taking care of people's needs and that Santa Claus will handle all of the sugarplum wishes for Christmas gifts and that somebody or something else will handle everything else.

Little kids don't think about things like food or heat or clothing. Those things just happen. I never thought about those things. When I began taking tap-dancing lessons, I had no reason to think that somebody must pay for these lessons. When it came time for my class to perform a recital, my innocent little mind had no reason to worry about who would pay for the dainty little outfit I'd wear during my few minutes on stage. Sears, J.C. Penney, Montgomery Wards, they all had catalogs, and many mining families shopped via catalog. My recital outfit came from one of these catalogs. Then I had no reason to think about where the dollars came from to pay for my recital outfit. It was so simple then, you picked out what you wanted and your mom mailed in some sort of form and it arrived eventually.

It was just like Christmas when all of those wonderful packages came in the mail.

It never occurred to me that Sears, "Monkey Wards," or the others required money for their wares. When you are little, everything is magic. Only when you become an adult yourself do you realize the hardships and sacrifices your parents have made to make the moments happen.

2

Right Of Imminent Domain

My early growing-up years went through many stages, just like any other kid. One day I might be involved with my crewcut baby dolls and imaginary friends...and the next I might be into rabbits! RABBITS! I didn't even know how or why I got into rabbit parenting, but I did, indeed, begin to raise rabbits. A shed behind our house gave home to my latest, serious project.

Yes, rabbits do tend to reproduce quite rapidly, and I quickly became the "mother" of around forty rabbits. Each with a name personally selected by me. I was serious about my project. Every morning I would get up early and go to the shed to feed my family. Many people like the taste of rabbit meat. Many do not. The point is mute, because I never began raising my family to fill the stomachs of humans. Most of my "kids" simply died of old age.

Bruiser was one of my favorites. A fuzzy buck who finally went to "rabbit heaven", perhaps, for the lack of anything better to do. My three brothers, by this time, had given up on turning my baby dolls into Ken dolls, but they hadn't given up on their oneryness. The night that Bruiser went to rabbit heaven, there was a special meat treat for supper, rabbit. At the supper table I was somewhat of a trooper about the coincidence until I was pushing the meat around my plate with a fork, one of my brothers piped up with, "Boy, doesn't Bruiser taste good!" I could have thrown up! Did Mom actually fry Bruiser? Needless to say, I ate mostly vegetables that night.

When you are a little kid growing up, especially in a rural setting, Christmas, and the events leading up to the big day are so special. Like many other country kids, I remember those times with a special fondness. The excitement. The secrets. The big day when you'd actually get to go into town and spend your two or three dollar hoard on gifts for the family. On a given day, depending on when Dad was off work, we would all plop into the family vehicle and go Christmas shopping. Boswell, as I realize now, was not a metropolis, but when you're just a farm kid, going into Boswell to shop, or for any reason, is an event in itself. When we annually went to Boswell for the purpose of Christmas shopping, it was a big event for all of us, especially me.

Once our family jalopy was parked, Dad would say, "OK kids, I'll meet you back here in two hours," and with that, we four offspring would go on our secret treasure hunts! How wonderful it was in those days that our parents did not have to be worried about us being molested or childnapped in Boswell. It wasn't so important what you bought each person. It was important that we could stare at an object long enough to convince one's self that it was the "right" gift for your loved one. It might only be a little plastic toy car for a brother, or a cheap folding fan for Mom, but the thrill for me was taking my pocketful of coins and turning it into gifts for Mom, Dad and my three cantankerous brothers. As I look back now, it's a wonder my Mom didn't end up with the little plastic car, my Dad with the folding fan, and at least one brother with a paring knife or a bottle of Evening In Paris perfume!

Once the treasures were bought, the rondezvous took

place and the family headed home, the excitement continued. When you've spent your little fortune on gifts, there's nothing left for store-bought wrappings, so you resort to encasing those treasures in scraps of butcher paper or even old newspapers. The frills seemed less important back then. Too bad it isn't that way today!

When you grow up in such simple Lutheran faith surroundings, there is no conflict between Santa Claus and Jesus Christ. You are celebrating the birthday of Jesus Christ with gifts provided by Santa, period! When you pray your childhood "Now I lay me down to sleep" prayer, you are talking to God and Jesus. But when it comes to celebrating Christ's birthday, you hope for presents which a jolly fat man in a red and white suit will deliver sometime after you've fallen asleep on the eve of Jesus' birthday. And, Christmas morning, it all wonderfully happens, and there's never reason to question it when you're little, just like there's no reason to question the sleepy look or dark circles beneath the eyes of your parents!

Now, a lot of people have artificial Christmas trees and store-bought decorations. Part of the thrill of the Christmas season for me was making decorations and stringing popcorn a few days before the big day. If you've never tried to stick a needle and thread through stubborn kernels of popcorn, you have no way of knowing how quickly little thumbs can become tender. The more seasoned popcorn kernel stringer will allow a batch of popped corn to dry out before attempting to string it, but the zeal of little kids sometimes precludes this precaution. Sore, needle-poked thumbs or not, it was a highlight of my childhood memories!

Looking back now, I fondly chuckle in my mind at the reality of our sick-looking Christmas trees, draped to drooping with icicles, but then, seeing them for the first time on Christmas morning, they were always more glorious than the Grand Canyon, Niagara Falls or the splendor of anything else. In my adult mind, I now know that our Christmas trees were probably always something chopped down from the woods, or a left-over, last-minute discounted evergreen orphan that nobody else wanted on Christmas eve. In reality, Dad probably dragged this pathetic looking reject into the house after us kids were asleep, and cut branches here, and drilled holes there, and with a bunch of sweat, cussing, praying, wire and "icicles", transformed an evergreen reject into the most spectacular sight my three brothers and I had ever seen. Each Christmas morning had to be a new challenge for Dad and Mom!

Any kid knows how long Christmas Eve can be. You have to go to bed long before you're sleepy, and stay awake longer than you would on any other night of the year. Forcing yourself to stay awake even after the sandman tries to tell you it's time to go to sleep is difficult, but you are determined to hear the sleigh bells, or hear those runners touch down on snow covered roofs.

There's always a plate of cookies and glass of milk on the table for Santa. Considering the millions of houses he must visit between the time the world's kids go to sleep and awake three hours later, it's no wonder he's so fat! But a child never thinks about these things. It's all enchantment, and it's that illusion in the mind of a child which makes Christmas so exciting.

On Christmas morning, children universally want to stay home and play with the toys that Santa has deposited under the tree for them. Any child know the AGONY of having to give into family ritual, of going to visit relatives on Christmas Day. You've stayed awake late; gotten up early; discovered the new treasures that Santa has left you, and now must be uprooted to go and spend this special day looking at somebody else's tree and treasures. It's a bummer, but tradition, so you abandon your new gifts, plop into the family car, and because of tradition go to Dad's sister's place in Berlin, about 30 miles away. Thanksgiving dinner was always spent at our house, and Christmas was spent at the relatives in Berlin. What bothered my brothers Harold,

Ron and Terrry, and me, was that we couldn't take our new toys with us. Dad's sister had five kids of her own, and having NINE kids fight over their newfound treasures at the same time was just too much, so the rule was that the Coughenour kids leave their toys at home. What agony for me, but you didn't question tradition!

It was Christmas at my aunts, Thanksgiving with us, and Easter at Grandpa's house. Though it was difficult for the multitude of offspring, it was easy in one respect, for we always knew where we were going to be on these special days. It wasn't until I was about 12 that Harold, Ron, Terry and I began to rebel against tradition, not that it did a lot of good. It didn't!

The house I was raised in was not a castle. It was "home" and it was our security; our world. The mine company didn't own it, it was our home, a modest dwelling to say the most. The house was cold in winter, with the thinnest wood walls and no insulation (that was unheard of then), but what we enjoyed or endured was ours, until one day when a man wearing a suit came to call.

When you live in a world of linoleum-covered floors and coal-fired heat stove, you never see somebody in a suit knocking at your door unless it's the preacher coming to call on Sunday afternoon, or someone concerning a funeral or wedding. But a stranger wearing a suit DID come calling unannounced, and shattered our security!

"Have you ever heard of the Right of Imminent Domain?" the stranger asked Dad. Dad said, "Well yes, but why?" (The Right of Imminent Domain is what the government uses when they need something which belongs to you.) In this case, the Commonwealth of Pennsylvania wanted to put a big highway right smack-dab through the middle of our farm. Granted the "state" (or, in this case, the "Commonwealth") would pay them, but the bottom line was that the Coughenour clan had to vacate their land before four months had passed. We four kids didn't know what "The Right Imminent

Domain" meant, but Dad and Mom knew, and it had to have been a crushing blow to their feeling of security.

If you go today to the site where our little dwelling once stood, there's no indication that it ever existed. There's nothing now but concrete and cars passing unknowingly over the gravesite of what was once our homestead. It's called "progress", and it often displaces dreams and shatters security. Dad was the "Rock of Girbralter". Nothing really ever upset him, but this change of events did. He was angry, and rightfully so, and depressed, probably rightfully so, and just plain mad! He was raised to be the head of the household; the bread winner; the source of security for his brood, and that had all been swept from beneath his feet in a matter of minutes. Oh, the Commonwealth of Pennsylvania thought they were fair, but Dad, as a DP offspring, now found his family in a Displaced Persons status, and it went againt the grain of everything his family had come to the new land, America, to avoid ever again. America is the land of opportunity, not displacement, but the edict from the State was cut and dry, and quite legal. VACATE YOUR PROPERTY, for it now belongs to the government.

Once Dad faced the reality of the situation, perhaps he managed to get the last lick after all. He was determined not to let his material life go up in a puff of dust without a "fitten" burial. The old farmhouse became a giant tombstone of sorts, as Dad and Mom invited their immediate family and close friends who had shared happy times there to sign their names and parting thoughts all over the walls of the house. The adults may have inscribed their notations more solemnly, but for us kids it was like Christmas out of season, because we were allowed to write all over the walls of the nearly deceased homestead after having been instructed that you never write on walls! When the walls finally did come tumbling down, they were filled with tributes from many people who had shared many happy hours within their confines.

If you drove down that sprawling highway now, you

would never know when you car passed over the spot where our house once stood. It was somewhere 40 feet below the massive mountain of dirt of the new highway. It is only a part of memory now. But Dad's memory will never forget that day his house came crashing down in what seemed to be nothing more than seconds. One minute the house which had provided shelter for dozens of seasons was standing, and the next minute it was a pile of ruins. It was one of the few times I ever remember my dad with tears in his eyes. Part of his heart died that day, but what made it hurt even more was once the culmination of his adult efforts had been reduced to a dusty pile of ruins, they set fire to what remained. It was like seeing a healthy living loved one die and be cremated, realizing that the small pile of ashes was all that remained of what once was!

Our family, our belongings, and livestock were moved to a farm a few miles away from the homestead gravesite, but no amount of money could ever pay for the loss which goes deeper than dollars. Memories are built; they can never be bought, and no amount of money can bring back what has been taken away.

The initial move from the old farm involved a lot of packing but only a short move, to a rented farm near Davidsville, just a few miles away. We were no sooner settled down and unpacking multitudes of cardboard boxes and crates, when we found out we had to move again. The man we were renting from died suddenly, and the caretaker of his estate wanted the farm back. So we were uprooted again, and again, until finally we were in our own home again, one which was built, in part, from the money paid us by the State for the initial displacement. Mom and Dad didn't get enough money to replace the farm, so they once again were in debt.

If it hadn't been for a simple, deep-rooted faith, Mom, Dad, my brothers and myself might never have adjusted to the moves or eventual settling into our new surroundings, but we did have faith and we did adjust.

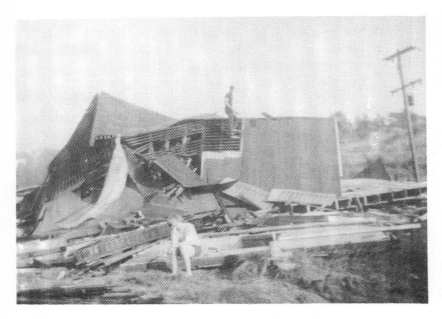

State destroys our house

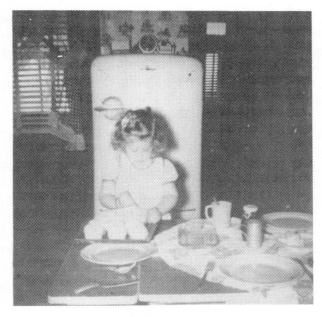

Patti, 3 years old

3

My New Friend

Church functions and holy holidays were special, you paid God the respect He deserved on such occasions. Each Sunday morning, Dad put on his suit and worn-out tie, Mom put on her Sunday best, the boys were not enthusiastic, but simply resolved themselves to dressing up and combing their hair, and I gladly put on the best I had. This may have been the only time during those years that I wouldn't rather be wearing jeans and hand-me-down shirts from my brothers. Sundays were always important to me. Any observation of an event which belonged to God was special to me. I really didn't know why, it just was.

Whether it was Easter, Christmas, or just going to church on Sunday, I always felt it was a special occasion, for God. In my small-town, small church upbringings, I was not exposed to a lot of church emotionalism. My country church was Lutheran. But, at a point, I simply knew that it was time to make a commitment on a deeper level to my God. Thus, I enrolled in catechism classes. Catechism is a series of classes which gives you a basic understanding of what, in an organized sense, your denomination believes. At my age, I didn't know that Catholics, Jews, Mennonites, Baptists, Methodists, Presbyterians, or hundreds of others also believed in a Supreme Being called God. All I knew was that I wanted to make a more serious commitment to the only God I knew from my upbringing, the Heavenly Father and the Father of Jesus.

It's odd that when you seek to know God on a deeper level, there always seem to be distractions, innocent circumstances which can lead you away from that deeper search. In my case it was the normal high school activities which would tempt any teenager. Wednesday night was catechism night at church. Yet, there were always these small temptations to distract me. One week it might be the peer pressure from my schoolmates to go to a basketball game or just another school buddy who wanted to do something that evening. There was probably a time in American history when nothing inter-fered with a church related function, but that time had long ago ceased to be. Now the burden was placed on the shoulders of the one who was determined to commit a greater part of their life to God.

For someone who has never been through catechism, it is not something which is taken lightheartedly; (at least for me it wasn't). It is taken seriously. Yes, it does have a lot to do with doctrinal positions, but is has as much or more to do with a personal commitment. It was that desire for personal commitment to God which led me to commit months and months of my life to these classes. The first two years of catechism I learned the Bible; Bible stories, the Apostles creed, Baptism, etc. I learned not only about communion, but what communion was all about when entered into seriously.

Entering the teen years, even without catechism, can be a rough experience even in the hills of Pennsylvania. At the same time your body is going through chemical changes which begin to prepare you for adulthood, your mind is bombarded by peers with new options. A commitment to my catechism classes meant that I would have to sacrifice a lot, because I was determined to approach a closer walk with God seriously. Had it not been for the true compassion and strength displayed by my country preacher, Pastor Clark, I may never had endured, but I did! I am the first one to give credit to a man obviously blessed by and filled with the Spirit of God.

Even before my decision to seek a deeper walk with God, I was greatly influenced by Pastor Clark's transparent Christian walk. He actually practiced and lived what he preached! What appeared to be simple faith on the surface came from a deeper source of power, and I wanted to know that Power in my life. The pastor always tried to instill a very uncomplicated faith and trust in the minds and hearts of his parishioners, because Pastor Clark simply believed that's how it worked, and that's how he preached and practiced.

Pastor Clark had neither a watered-down or hyped-up faith. It's as transparent as a fine crystal goblet. You can see the outside, but there's no problem seeing what's inside either. When it came to having a hand in helping to develop the minds of young people, Pastor Clark was firm without being pushy beyond our ability to comprehend. A simple faith, rising from a deeper stream of strength, was always stressed.

A girl just entering puberty, according to psychological experts, is far more emotionally advanced than her male counterpart, but very few are making serious plans about choosing a lifelong mate. Yet, Pastor Clark impressed on the younger members of his flock, both boys and girls, to earnestly pray for a good husband or wife. The Bible states that people shouldn't be unevenly yoked. Whether in friendships, business relationships or, most important, in marriage. As less and less consideration has been given to this truth, more and more divorces have resulted. The parting line in a modern divorce is, "We have nothing in common." Maybe that's what Pastor Clark was trying to get us young people to think about. The Bible may be speaking in totally spiritual terms, but the truth of being unevenly yoked, if applied, could spare many heartaches, disillusionments, and divorces in the non-Christian community as well! How can you seriously pray for a good lifetime mate at twelve or thirteen? You can't! But God doesn't analyze everything the way we do. He probably weighs the sincerity rather than the content of each of our prayers. So, I did pray that the Lord would bring the right partner into my life. It would be years before I realized that He had answered my special prayers.

Catechism may be a ritual of sorts, to some young people, but under the direction of Pastor Clark it involved a true commitment, and he didn't push any real leading of the Holy Spirit in each individual life. He had learned patience. He was willing to wait until we kids really understood what we were doing. Beneath the pageantry of the Lutheran faith, the pastor knew there had to be an individual commitment to the center of the pageantry, Jesus Christ! That commitment, Pastor Clark knew, had to come from God Himself. For the preacher, it was like planting seeds and then patiently watching for the tiny sprouts to reach heavenward and innocently open up to a food that only the sun could provide.

Confirmation is the ceremonial climax of weeks and months of dedication to catechism classes. That ritual would not take place with Pastor Clark until everybody was in unison. If there were those who didn't fully understand, he was willing to wait. He would make the entire group wait until the last one truly understood. My particular group of catechism faithfuls had to wait several weeks until Pastor Clark knew that the entire flock knew what they knew, and why.

Even after he was sure, this dear man took each of us to the altar and prayed individually with each one. When he felt in his heart that each had accepted Jesus Christ as our personal Savior, he knew the flock was ready to be confirmed into the faith.

I had always known there was a God, and had been raised with true Godly values, but it wasn't until confirmation that I really found Jesus Christ. The denominational label doesn't get a person to heaven. Somehow, at some point, I knew that. I didn't know how I knew, I just knew. Being raised in a Christian home doesn't make you a Christian; going to church every Sunday doesn't make you a Christian; receiving a pin or a New Testament for perfect attendance in Sunday school doesn't make you a Christian. Somewhere deep down inside my almost teenage being, I somehow knew that.

There were probably those in my catechism group to whom it didn't have a real spiritual meaning. Maybe God's Holy Spirit had not yet tapped them on the spiritual shoulder. Through those long months, the denominational literature and study guides had exposed truths to us. Pastor Clark had done his best to go beyond the printed words to lead us to that deeper level. But, in individual lives, only God could make it really happen. For me, that happened at Confirmation.

The Lutheran denomination, an offshoot of the Catholic church, is a faith filled with pageantry, beautiful pageantry. Especially during the most sacred "high holidays" of the Christian faith. But it was not pageantry which I accepted. It was Jesus Christ, the center of the celebration.

At this point in my life, I had not yet been exposed to other denominations. I was naive to the conflicts going on within the Christian faith. I believe in the doctrines of the Lutheran denomination, and now know how misunderstood those doctrines are, not unlike the doctrines of Catholics, Baptists, Mennonites, Pentecostals, Methodists, Presbyterians, or a multitude of others. It may be a sad commentary to a lost and dying world that we, the different denominations, seem to be at such odds with each other. In later years, this bothered me. While the outside world was, and is, searching for the true answer, they may be being bombarded with choosing a denomination rather than Jesus Christ Himself. Within each Christian denomination, where is Jesus Christ? To those who are searching, both inside and outside any denomination, the answer to that question is eternally critical.

As I grew in years and spiritual maturity, I began to appreciate my Lutheran faith and it hurt me that those outside of my beliefs didn't understand what Martin Luther or his rebellion were all about. Sometimes the most blood is shed on the true Christian battlefield by Christians wounding other Christians. The outside world watches, rightfully bewildered or skeptical.

Martin Luther never intended that people should follow him as a Messiah. Even though some probably did and do. His rebellion was not against God, but against a form of religious politics which had, in his mind, dethroned Jesus Christ as the center of His church. Since Martin Luther's rebellion over 500 years ago, many denominations have popped up in the same way; out of, for the most part, a holy rebellion at lukewarmness toward the center of true faith. In these offshoots, both individual egos and misunderstanding have taken their toll.

When I finally grew in years and discovered that there was a faith other than Lutheran, I learned secondhand about the others. I heard that all Baptists were stiff and stuffy, that all Pentecostals would swing from the rafters and jump and shout during their services and sometimes even pass out on the floor. How disrespectful in "God's House!" But I also painfully discovered that many in the Christian circle thought that all Lutherans simply followed some antiquated church ritual without being really "saved!" I began to realize that most of the blood shed on the Christian battlefield is caused by misunderstanding within the denominational community. And most of the bloodshed has nothing to do with the blood shed by Jesus Christ for all of us.

At confirmation, through a touch of God's Holy Spirit, I knew what and in Whom I believed. I knew that there

were Christian and non-Christian Lutherans, Mennonites, Baptists, Pentecostals, Methodists,
Presbyterians, Church of God, Church of Christ, and on
down the list. Without Jesus Christ, His virgin birth,
His death and resurrection, there is no faith. Regardless
of denominational label, without accepting and receiving
Him, one might as well spend Sunday morning in bed as
in a denominational religious assembly. Powerful words,
but true.

While Martin Luther was the founder of the
denomination, I knew that Jesus Christ was and is the
foundation of the faith. Through my studies, I became
deeply inspired by Martin Luther. One voice crying out
in the wilderness, daring to stand up and say, "No, it is
not idols that save us, it is grace. HERE I STAND!"
The grace of God through the shed blood of His Son,
Jesus Christ. He lashed out at the institution the
Catholic church of his day had become. He was not
against his beloved Catholic church. He was against
what she had become, and for his convictions he was
excommunicated.

There were those who began to follow Luther, to raise
him up as some great prophet. Others even placed him
right up there with God and Jesus. He rejected that, for
it was that sort of idolatry which he had fought within
his Catholic church. Then his band of followers thought
it would please Luther if they went into the churches and
smashed the idols and statues. Things got very much
out of hand with his zeal-filled band of followers. Martin
Luther never intended there to be a Lutheran church. He
was not breaking away in order to start another
denomination. At that point there was only one. He was
simply trying to show the mother church that without
grace, there is no true Christian church. In that his
became the second denomination, and there are today
hundreds, if not thousands. It would appear that the
echo of his long silent voice cries in the wilderness even
now.

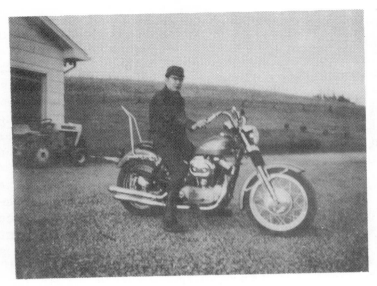

"My Prince"

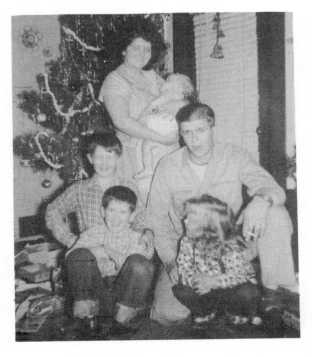

Mom holding Terry
Harold, Ron, Dad and me

4

My Prince

I was now Confirmed. I had been accepted into the small Lutheran fold and had personally accepted Jesus Christ into my heart, to lead me as I began my walk through this earthly life. I had made the biggest commitment of my life, and I was only thirteen.

Kathy was my very best friend. We were inseparable. Perhaps she was the sister I had always wanted. When you're only thirteen, you can't talk to your mother about the fears and frustrations which rush through your mind, and you sure can't talk to any of three brothers who still insisted on treating you as a kid! Kathy and I shared our secrets about boys, or a cute student teacher who made our pulse race a little faster. If I ever did mention a heartthrob to my brothers, they would go into hysterics and then tell me everything that was wrong with the kid.

I wanted the leading of God's Holy Spirit in my early frustrations with boys, but figured the Holy Spirit certainly didn't need the help of my three ornery brothers!

Weeks became months; months turned into seasons, and I continued to survive my teen years. I became more involved in school activities, and Kathy and I continued to share our frustrations of growing up.

When I was sixteen, or not many months shy, my brother Ron brought a buddy home. His name was Frank. I thought he was O.K., but didn't think he was serious when he eventually asked me for a date. He was twenty-two, and after all I was only sixteen. At later points in life, such a small age difference means nothing, but when you're only sixteen and only a sophomore in high school, and he's already a man of the world, that's a different story.

A big night was coming up, the banquet to wrap up the football season. I had been in the marching band all season and was looking forward to the gala evening. There was also a boy I was really interested in seeing there. We palled around together quite a bit. The guy probably thought of me as a buddy, but my feelings for him went much deeper, and I was excited about sharing such an important evening with him.

Not many days before the banquet, Frank again asked me for a date. That was his second request, and my second denial. My buddy/boyfriend was going to be there, and even though we weren't going to the banquet together, I didn't want to mess up a chance to be with him.

With the passage of time, the tomboy part of me took a back seat to the more feminine attributes which were surfacing. I spent hours preparing for the banquet, making sure my clothing looked just right, and I made several visits to the mirror to make certain each hair was in place. I wanted to look right for him, just in case he should notice me. The thought of giving up such a special occasion to go for a ride on Frank's motorcycle seemed preposterous! He was probably just kidding around anyway.

As the evening wore on, it may have seemed less and less preposterous, for my heartthrob spent the entire evening talking to another girl. The banquet was held in the fire hall in Jerome. My ego was somewhat dented, for

I spent the whole evening sitting alone, watching my buddy/boyfriend having a wonderful time on the other side of the room. At some point Frank drove by the firehouse on his cycle. I hoped he didn't notice how miserable I was, and also mentally kicked myself in the seat for turning down a bona fide date, for a fantasy which would obviously become nothing more.

It must have been the third or fourth time that Frank asked me out that I finally accepted. I learned much later that if I had rejected him that time, he had determined he would not ask again. Frank was the only male my brothers ever gave approval to. Maybe it was because Ron had introduced us. Yes, there was an age difference, but my brothers liked Frank. My brothers, though always playing pranks on me in earlier years, became very protective of me once I started noticing the difference between boys and girls. Because Frank was Ron's buddy, maybe the brothers-three knew I would be "safe" with him. After all, they're not getting married, just a few innocent dates!

Our first date was nothing more than a ride on Frank's motorcycle. We zig-zagged down narrow roads etched into the Pennsylvania countryside. I was not used to riding on a two-wheeled machine with nothing to hold onto. The sheer will to survive led my thumbs to the loops in Frank's jeans. I was just too shy to wrap my arms around his midriff, but had sense enough to know that if I didn't hold onto some part of him, he'd be riding solo in very short order!

The dates which followed were very simple by more cosmopolitan standards: cycle rides in the country; bowling, things like that. We were both athletic and loved the outdoors. It wasn't long before we each realized we also loved one another.

Dad and Mom accepted Frank. Like the brothers-three, they considered me their little girl, and wanted to protect me from the hurts of life, but also knew they had to let go. In "letting go," I always knew that they would be there when I needed them.

My paremts saw the love between Frank and me. They knew eventually Frank would approach them with a question which would change their little girl's life. Their values were very traditional, and they raised us children to respect those values too. If love was real, and the commitment was deep, you didn't just run off and live together. You even asked permission to be engaged. That special day finally arrived.

"But you're a different religion," Dad said, in response to Frank's asking permission to be engaged to me. "No problem," Frank shot back with no hesitation. "I'll change to Lutheran." He was a member of the Catholic church, but was not devoted or committed to his denomination. If Frank loved their little girl that much, Mom and Dad knew they had to give their blessing.

I was a senior when Frank asked me to marry him, so it was quite a special Christmas. Of course, Christmas at the Coughenour house was always special, but this one stood out in my mind as being, in many ways, the beginning of my life.

When Frank and I began dating regularly, many of my school friends couldn't understand what I saw in him, an "older" man. Even my best friend Kathy remarked several times, "But, he's so old." Through the eyes of a seventeen-year-old, he probably was, but through my eyes of love, I saw my life's mate, and nobody would discourage our mutual love.

When word got around school that Christmas season that Frank and I were engaged, many of my classmates fully expected to see my stomach begin to expand shortly with child. It was the only reason they could figure that I would marry this older man. Time obviously proved their suspicions totally wrong.

We both loved the rolling Pennsylvania hills. Frank appreciated the tomboy side of me. It allowed us to enjoy mutually spending hours outdoors roaming the countryside in search of wild life during the hunting season. I was a good squirrel hunter, maybe too good as far as my, then, boyfriend was concerned. Having been raised with three brothers, I learned how to handle firearms with respect at a young age. I also learned to handle a rifle or shotgun with considerable accuracy, so by the time Frank and I were roaming the hills in search of squirrels, it was not uncommon for me to get my limit in no time, while Frank would bag only one or two.

Frank also enjoyed trap shooting. Little clay discs are released from a spring-loaded device. The object is to shoot them out of the sky before they hit the ground. I always went trap shooting with Frank, but would never actually shoot at the clay pigeons myself. Even in my somewhat tomboy mind, it just wasn't ladylike! Besides, I enjoyed reloading his shotgun shells, and especially watching my future husband having fun doing something at which he was very good.

In many ways, I had placed Frank on a pedestal. He was my hero, my protector, friend and love. I found great pleasure in just being with him, and watching him be himself. Maybe because he was older in my young eyes, I always thought Frank could solve any problem. I felt secure with him and knew he would never betray that trust.

Not long after our engagement, we were invited by my oldest brother Ron and his wife to go hunting with them at White Horse Mountain, a short distance from our farm. Ron and his wife were recently married and thought it would be nice to spend the day with us doing something we all enjoyed. Dad had a cabin at White Horse Mountain. Just a shack really with no modern conveniences. It was in the dead of winter, so we decided to use the cabin for shelter that day. There was no way to get there other than via a maze of dirt roads and trails.

It was a threatening looking day and better judgment would have prodded us to put off the day in the wilderness until another time. We were young and adventuresome, and looking forward to the outing, so we went, figuring that if it began to snow we could simply head home. No problem. However, we didn't count on

one of those snowstorms which comes out of nowhere.
One minute, just cloudy skies, and the next minute we
couldn't even see the sky due to the wall of snow which
had materialized.

Ron and Brenda figured they could weather out the
storm in the relative safety of the cabin. They had some
food and had no cause for concern. Even though there
was no phone, Mom and Dad knew where we were and
would realize what happened when we didn't return
home that evening. Dad knew that both Ron and Frank
were seasoned outdoorsmen and could keep Brenda and
me safe. Frank was in agreement with Ron and Brenda,
but I wouldn't hear of it. Blizzard or not, we were going
home, that very night.

What would it look like if Frank and I spent the night
together in that cabin? What would Mom and Dad
think? I held my folks in such high esteem and I couldn't
bear the thought that they might be angry with me if
Frank and I spent the night together in the cabin. So the
two men went out into the storm and spent hours
breaking a path which would allow them to escape to
civilization or, in particular, the Coughenour homestead.
Frank grumbled as he and Ron labored in the snow-
storm, but he respected me and my respect for Mom and
Dad. It was a night none of us would forget, and years
later, could all laugh about.

Frank and I didn't argue much. If we grumbled about
anything, it was that sometimes little details irritated
me and nothing seemed to bother Frank. When I would
get fumed about something, Frank would just say in his
soft mumble, "Oh, Patti you fuss too much. It's not
important." When I was upset about something, maybe
Frank's calm predictable response irritated me more
than my current irritation! He was just easy-going by
nature, and nothing ever bothered him. I couldn't
understand that and quite often misread it as not caring.

At one point before our marriage though, I would not
budge on a point. I was determined not to give in to
Frank's indifference. Frank was a truck and motorcycle

man. To him, a handsome machine looked "macho". Not that he was into any male ego trip. He simply liked trucks and bikes and could care less about owning a car, no matter how "macho" it looked or how many horses were crammed under the hood.

My senior prom was approaching and I wanted everything to be just right. Any tomboy inclinations within me gave way totally to any girl's dream for her prom night: the gown, dainty shoes, corsage and her date picking her up wearing a suit and driving a well-polished car. Frank didn't go in for formal gatherings. He had consented to shackle himself with a suit and tie because he knew it was important to me, but he couldn't understand why I was making such a fuss about his picking me up in his truck! "No way am I crawling into a truck with my gown on and everything," I fumed. Frank couldn't understand me fussing over such a little thing, but figured if it was that important, he'd borrow his brother-in-law's car for the evening. So we went to the prom in style. Frank was miserable, but I enjoyed my special evening!

Just two months after saying goodbye to high school days forever, Frank and I were married. From graduation until the August wedding, I was busy making plans for that day above all days in a young girl's life.

In early July we began looking for our first home. We had both agreed that a mobile home would be most practical, so spent a lot of our free time looking at trailers. If you've never walked through a series of mobile homes with their varying floor plans, furniture and features, you can't grasp my excitement. My background was traditional. Our home was comfortable, but I was used to hand-me-downs. Trying to choose something which was entirely new, from the carpeting to the toilet bowl, was a new experience for me. I was like Alice in Wonderland. We finally decided on a mobile home which had the floor plan, furnishings, and features we liked. From my standpoint it was a mansion and Frank was my prince.

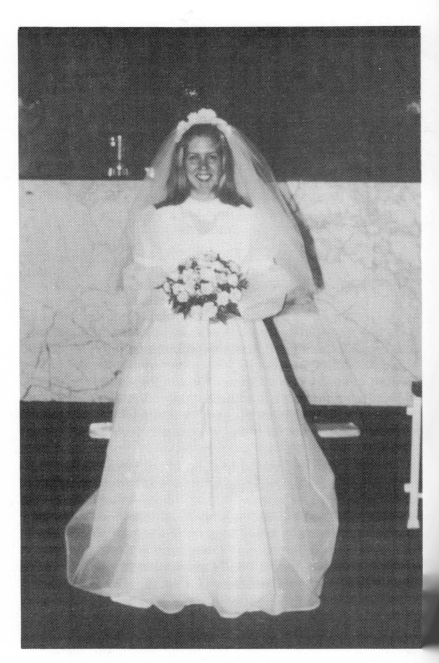

My Penny's Gown

5

My Penny's Gown

Perhaps my parents accepted my impending marriage because they knew that Frank wasn't simply a high school infatuation. Yes, he was older than their little girl, but he was also less flighty than my male high school peers. He had a job and more than the shirt on his back, and seemed determined to take care of their only female offspring, and that comforted Mom and Dad. Then too, they knew that Frank's parents (even though Polish Catholics) had the same protective attitude regarding their son and future daughter-in-law.

The homesite for our new portable mansion would be in the yard of my life-long neighbors. They had through the years become like another set of parents to me. Frank and I already had our mobile home set up there, so it was all so practical, the water, sewage and electricity were already hooked up. All had agreed on a monthly rent for the space and hook-up once our mansion was moved to the site.

Frank and I were more fortunate than many couples entering into marriage, for we already had our brand new home with all new furnishings awaiting us.

To say the least at that point I had forgotten that I had prayed to God for my lifemate, but God hadn't forgotten! In retrospect, I can now begin to realize this. We were so opposites in so many ways. Even when shopping for the trailer, I was the impulsive one while Frank was the exact opposite. As a result, during our shopping sprees, it was common for me to fall in love with the first mobile home we walked through, while Frank was always so non-committal. We would spend hours on a Saturday driving within a 100 mile radius on his motorcycle just visiting mobile home sales lots! Miles back I had decided on the home I wanted, I think it was the first one we toured, but Frank wanted to shop around more and then some more. I didn't understand it at the time, but it could be attributed, in most part, to my immaturity. Our first "mansion" was much more the result of Frank's patience than my maturity or common sense at that point.

Mom and I had to be very creative in the wedding plans. Dad, being a practical man, had set a limit on the wedding expenses. It may only seem like a drop in the bucket now, but his $500 limit was then quite liberal, considering my parents' modest means. I would have loved a bridal gown out of Vogue or some other fashion magazine, but that would have shot Dad's allotment for the entire wedding and reception. Mom and I had to put our creative minds to work.

Every teenage bride-to-be wants a one of a kind bridal gown. One created for her alone. We couldn't afford that, and that was that! Mom and I searched the catalogs, Wards, Sears and J.C. Penny. J.C. Penny won our pauper's search for a non-exclusive, "exclusive" wedding gown. I was searching the catalogs for the best alternative to a handmade gown, but Mom was searching for a factory-made gown that she could doctor up, to look exclusive! The gown finally arrived at the Penny catalog store in Johnstown, about 17 miles away from our home. The mail-order gown only cost $60, a respectable price then. Once the gown arrived at the

Johnstown Penny's store, Mom and I drove into the metropolis to claim our treasure. Whether it comes from a mail-order house or not, it is a special event for any young girl to take possession of her very own wedding gown. Mom and I shared the mutual electricity of the event. The garment we picked up that day was a far cry from what I wore as I walked down the aisle on my wedding day. What Mom eventually created for me from that mail-order gown resulted in a one-of-a-kind designer's creation. I don't think that Christian Dior could have designed a more excellent wedding gown. What Mom did to that Penny gown would have even impressed Rembrant, Dior or Laurent.

As any former bride knows though, the gown is only one part of a very big ceremony. When I began to total my list of invitations to be sent, it became apparent that the number of people greatly outnumbered the capacity of my small Lutheran church to accommodate those people, should they all decide to attend the wedding ceremony! Since my church in Jerome could only handle 50-60 people then, it was decided that the ceremony would be performed at a larger Lutheran church in Davidsville, a short distance away. It was agreed that Pastor Clark, my pastor, would officiate the ceremony.

I wanted a morning wedding, so that's what we had. The church in Davidsville was a bit foreign, to me, but it accommodated my needs and desires. The Davidsville church had beautiful stained-glass windows, and the morning sunlight bathed the sanctuary in a holy awesome beauty. I was really pleased.

A formal wedding is, in many respects, like a play, because what the spectator sees on the wedding day is the result of practice and rehearsals! You have to go through practice runs before the actual ceremony. More often than not the rehearsal goes without flaw, but the actual wedding can be a chain-reaction "comedy of errors"!

"Are the pants to my tuxedo at the house?" It was Ron's voice, my brother, on the other end of the telephone. I was already a nervous bride-to-be and had enough problems of my own, and couldn't believe that my brother, the older...and wiser offspring, could bother me just minutes before the ceremony with such a trivial question. Ron might have been the older offspring, but NOT the most personally organized. I was so involved in simply getting married, that I could have cared less whether or not Ron wore his pants or not in the wedding party! Sure I would have been embarrassed, but how dare him to have misplaced his pants at the last minute! Oh, how I love that precious brother of mine.

As the minutes clicked away, I became less concerned with whether or not Ron found his pants, as to whether or not Frank would make it to the church on time. Even though in a traditional marriage the bride and groom are not supposed to see each other prior to the ceremony, I became increasingly concerned that I would be the only one standing before Pastor Clark at the altar.

"Is Frank here yet?" I asked again and again. In my upbringing, I was taught promptness and as the seconds ticked away before my wedding ceremony, I was becoming more and more worried that Frank had not also been raised to respect promptness. How could I dare to walk down the aisle of this foreign, but beautiful, sanctuary alone not knowing if Frank would be there to make the ceremony complete.

Frank was notoriously late in our relationship, but this was too much. I couldn't imagine his being late for his own wedding. We had talked about all of these things long before the wedding, or rehearsal. It is supposed to be the guy who does the waiting in a relationship, but in my case it was the other way around. When we were dating, I was always ready at the agreed time, only to have to wait for Frank's late arrival. He has since learned promptness, but back then his constant lateness was the cause of much irritation for me, as was his, "Aw honey, you fuss too much" response.

Ron managed to find his pants, and Frank managed to find the church and the wedding ceremony sailed along without a snag. I had attended enough weddings to know that I didn't want my groom to have that look of agony which most grooms wear as the bride makes her way down the aisle. "When I walk down the aisle, Frank, you smile. I don't care what you are feeling inside, you smile! You must do this for me, please," I pleaded. As this eighteen year old nervously made my way down the aisle, Frank was wearing the most beautiful smile I had ever seen. It was probably that reassuring smile of my groom which kept my legs from turning to Jello.

The ceremony was beautiful. Unbeknownst to me, my mother had hidden a tape recorder on the altar behind a spray of flowers. A year later, Mom gave us the recording as our first anniversary gift. What a wonderful and precious gift.

Most newlyweds only have to endure one wedding reception. But Frank and I had two. Since many of my friends were of the Mennonite faith, I wanted them to have a reception at which they could feel comfortable. In that we had a morning wedding, the first reception was a simple luncheon, cold cuts, sandwiches, potato salad and soft drinks. However, since Frank's family is Polish, the second reception was a bit more lively, not an old country drinking bash, but still with a lot more spirit, and spirits, than my Mennonite friends could have handled.

A Polish wedding reception is an event, and ours was no exception. There was a big sit-down meal at a big hotel restaurant, complete with wine, dancing, and a good time was had by all. Frank is a Levi's man, and being trapped inside a tuxedo was murder for him. Even as we were sitting down to eat, he was whispering to me, "Hurry up, I want to get out of here." Maybe it was the engine roars at the stock car races across from the hotel which were tempting Frank to escape. The Polish reception may very well have gone on into the wee hours, but as most newlyweds do, Frank and I disappeared at some point, but at that point, most of the well-wishers were so involved in celebrating the event rather than the couple, that few probably noticed our departure.

Our escape vehicle was Frank's truck with his motorcycle in the enclosed bed. No fancy car, just a truck, but that was Frank and I had accepted him just the way he was. During the reception, some of the kids had decorated the vehicle in traditional garb, with newlywed slogans written in white shoe polish. I thought it was cute. Frank as usual didn't say anything. Our immediate destination was Frank's parents' home where we both escaped the confines of our costumes. Frank gladly traded his tux for denim. Of course I being modest, went into the privacy of Frank's parents' bedroom and changed from my gown into my travelling clothes. Once we were ready, we took our luggage, got into the truck and hit the road. We drove and drove and eventually ended up in New York state. By today's standards, I am certain that I would be considered quite old-fashion and square. I was TERRIFIED of my wedding night.

Sure, Frank and I had kissed, hugged and held hands while we were going together, and perhaps our deeper passions were aroused at times, but "fooling around" was just not an option in our pre-marital relationship. And now, here we were on our wedding night. Each mile brought us closer to our eventual honeymoon motel room. As the miles to that destination decreased, my fears increased! I had no regrets for keeping myself pure for my new husband. That did not alter the fact that I was still scared.

Frank was, and is, a down to earth wonderful guy. No real hang-ups. When we finally arrived at the motel, he couldn't really understand my nervousness or snappy responses to his conversation. But bless his heart, he had already learned to accept me, as is, also. When we walked into the motel room, all Frank wanted to do was kick off his boots and relax. All I saw was the bed! When Frank started unbuttoning his shirt to become more comfortable, I darted for the bathroom where I changed into my night clothes before hopping into the big bed, pulling the covers snugly around my shoulders. Frank was older, somewhat wiser, understanding, patient, and very loving...Yes, God had indeed sent me the husband of my prayers.

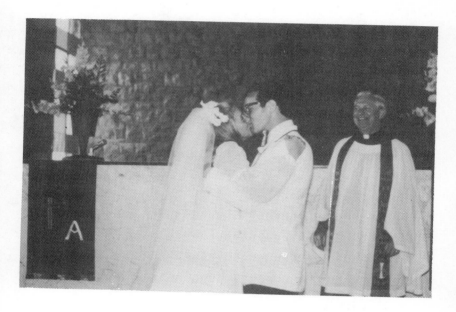

Pastor Clark appoves!

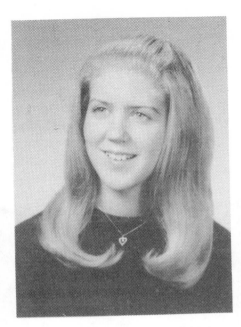

Patti, High School graduation

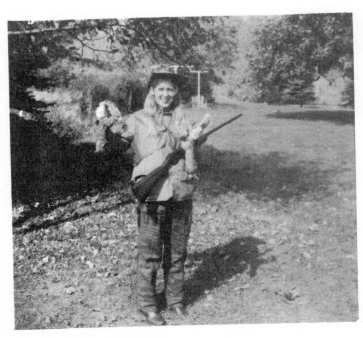

The Great Hunter

6

An Angel From God

Frank had very few days off for the honeymoon, so we quickly returned to our new home and began the routine of married life together. I had always wanted to be a nurse, and Frank had always encouraged me to pursue a career. Many schools required then that you remain single during your training and Frank, bless his heart, was even willing to postpone our wedding to enable me to go through my nurse's training. No way! I thought our marriage was more important than the marital requirements of a nursing school. From his standpoint, Frank didn't want me to harbour feelings of resentment 20-30 years down the road because I had sacrificed a career for marriage.

Once we moved into our 12 foot wide mobile home mansion, I found a one year practical nursing course which had no marital requirements, so a month after our marriage, I was again a student. Frank had already returned to school to become a licensed electrician before we were married. Had it not been for the money which his parents had set aside for his future, our mobile home, my nursing training or Frank's electrical schooling would not have been possible. Frank and I were both blessed with wonderful in-laws.

An eighteen year old never thinks of boredom which lies beyond the honeymoon, but it did arrive. When a couple are courting, every moment together is special. But when the courting ends and real life begins, it can be a rude awakening! Prior to my starting nursing school, I would see Frank off to work and then face eight or ten hours alone in our trailer home. Without children, there is nothing to occupy a new bride's time or mind. It was either a blessing or a curse that my Mom only lived about half-a-mile up the road, because I found myself driving or walking the short distance quite often, sometimes spending the whole day with my Mom, being sure to get home in time to fix Frank's supper.

Then school started and the routine turned from boredom to hectic. I went from not knowing what to do with my idle time, to having no idle time! My days were spent in classes. My nights were spent in books, studying for the next day's classes or tests. It was only natural that Frank would want to spend time with me, his bride after a hard day at work. After all, in our courtship I was always available, to go riding his cycle or stalking the woods in search of animal prey. Now that we were married, he wanted me with him all the more.

"But Frank, I have five chapters to read." "But hunner," his nickname for me, "you can bring your books and read while I hunt." Frank always made everything seem so simple and uncomplicated. Our first few months together in marriage, I entered nursing school and Frank entered deer hunting season. It wasn't that he wanted me to hunt with him, but simply that Frank wanted me in the field with him. Believe it or not, I would take my books and we would go out into the woods together. The thought of it is quite humorous, but Frank would find a stately-looking tree in the woods, and that would become my temporary study hall, not under it, but up in it! Frank would get me and books securely nestled in the embracing arms of a friendly tree, perhaps five or ten feet up (I was petrified of heights), and go off in search of deer. Eventually he would return, long after there was not enough light remaining to see the words on the printed page.

Frank kept insisting that I become a participant in his deer hunting expeditions. I had no problems with hunting squirrels, because they reminded me of rats. But when it came to shooting a deer, I could only think of my childhood Bambi stories. One day we went out deer hunting together. Frank was more aggressive and went into the bush hoping to steer a deer in my direction. He did! I took aim in my rifle sight. I knew that in order to score a hit on a running animal, you must sight ahead of your prey. I did, squeezed the trigger, and saw the animal stumble and fall. "Frank, oh, Frank!", I screamed. He came running, thinking that I had shot myself. "Are you hurt? What's the matter?" he yelled. "I hit it, I hit it," I hysterically replied. Frank was thrilled. I was heart-broken. I had killed a Bambi!! Believe me when I say, that was the last time I ever went big game hunting.

Perhaps Frank and I were spared many of the newlywed scraps, because we simply didn't see each other that much. Two people can really love each other in a dating, or courting situation, and still get on each other's nerves once they are thrown into a live-in marriage situation. With my schooling and study, and Frank's working 7-3, 3-11, or 11-7, our main form of communication in those early married days was via notes. That may have spared us many of the knit-picking squabble of most young married couples. Through inconvenience, we survived those early days together, because we were apart most of the time!

Minute by minute, the year of my training dragged, but in retrospect, it flew by and my graduation day arrived. It was my second meaningful ceremony in just over a year. Though there were only four blacks in my graduating class, none of the spectators had any problem spotting me in the graduating ensemble. As chance would have it, I ended up sandwiched between two of the four black students in my graduating class.

Mom and Dad were very proud of me. In a coal-mining rural community, very few offspring ever broke out of the blue-collar syndrome, especially female offspring. But I did it, I broke out of the mold and it didn't matter that I as a girl rather than one of their three male offspring, my parents were proud! You would have to understand the accepted oppressive blue-collar attitude of a coal-mining patch, to really appreciate what it really meant to Mom and Dad to see their little girl end up with a real profession.

After I graduated, there was still the state exam in Harrisburg to take. Several other classmates and I drove there together. We were all apprehensive. I came through with flying colors, and was finally certified by the Commonwealth of Pennsylvania to practice nursing. Frank was supportive, but just was not prone to show real enthusiasm, emotion or encouragement. I as a female had conquered many stereotype obstacles at that point. While Frank encouraged me to excel, he never knew how to show encouragement to me in those early years. He was glad for what I had done and accomplished, but did not seem very impressed! From my standpoint, I could not understand this coolness or apparent indifference. My nursing career aside, Frank and I had mutually agreed that we would have a baby. With Frank it was rather matter-of-fact. "We are going to make a baby, I hope it's a boy and that's that!" It didn't mean that Frank was uncaring, but simply that his upbringing conditioned him to be male blue-collar macho and very sure of himself.

When I finally discovered that I was pregnant, Frank was happy. In typical fashion, I first told my mother. Mom was thrilled that her only daughter was with child. They were probably all subconsciously hoping for a male child, but that never came up in conversation.

Whether pre or post sexual revolution, when you discover that you are pregnant and are not going to resort to the option of abortion, you must begin to consider names for the yet unborn child. For whatever reason, if it was a girl, I loved and chose the name Libby. Frank, on the other hand, said it sounded like a can of peaches. Names that Frank liked, male or female, I did not like. I probably had more names for an eventual little girl than a boy. The only name I came up with, should my baby be a boy, was Brett! "How", my friends asked, "did you come up with that name?" "I found it in a name book," was my calm reply. Maybe subconsciously, I wanted to name my first child after my mother, Betty. Maybe Brett was the closest I could come to Betty should I end up with a boy in the delivery room! A boy it was, and Brett he was!

How ironic that I should go into labor on Labor Day weekend, but I did, and labor, I did. 23-hours in labor! The last holiday of summer was always a big event for us Coughenours. It was the last family cook-out get-together of the summer season. Frank and I were there. At that point I was pregnantly miserable, but determined to attend the family gathering. Since the year before, there were many in attendance who had not yet met my new husband, let alone accept how close to the edge of child deliverance I was. I always enjoyed or endured the last family holiday of the summer season, but because I was a first-time mother-to-be, and feeling so miserable, I simply endured this particular family gathering in August of 1974.

Relatives I had not seen in years, or at least since the last Labor Day reunion, greeted the newest family member, Frank. Most of them congratulated me on the extended condition of my lower belly. Even though I was now twenty years old, I appreciated their well wishes, but also feared the unknown of my pregnant condition! I would sure be relieved when it was all over. As the clan enjoyed hamburgers, hotdogs and potato salad together, I began to experience more and more discomfort. Though I had no practical experience at child bearing, I suddenly knew that it was time.

At the Labor Day family reunion, I was determined not to let any of the clan know that I was going into labor simply because I didn't want the entire Labor Day celebration to follow me to the hospital! And I really believed they would. When I began to experience the first stages of labor pains, I knew it was getting close to delivery time. I motioned to Frank. He quickly responded and I asked him to quietly alert Mom. Thus, the time arrived and the three of us quietly exited for the local hospital, but not before I insisted that Frank go home and shave. I was going into labor, but I was determined that Frank would be clean-shaven at the arrival of our first child! Boy, I was tough to live with!

Once we arrived at the hospital, even the doctors and nurses kidded me about going into labor on Labor Day. They were trying to comfort me, but I found little comfort in my discomfort and their sick jokes. It became even more frustrating for me when I saw the same recycled cast of nurses almost a day later, and I had yet to deliver a baby!

After the final moments of my prolonged labor were ending, I was wheeled into the delivery room and, in short order, a male child was delivered. "A boy?", I mumbled. "Oh, Frank will be so happy!" The doctor looked down at me and questioned, "Aren't you happy too?" "Oh, yeah", I mustered, but it was really for Frank that I was thrilled. At that point, however, Brett was nothing more than a relief from my labor pains!

At birth, little Brett was a long, skinny thing. Twenty-one inches long, and only weighing six pounds, five ounces. Though it was hospital procedure to issue a card to relatives visiting the newborn nursery, so that the nurse would be sure to hold up the right baby, no card was necessary for young Brett's visitors. He was the only white baby in the entire nursery. It was comical when family would visit my room and then leave to go down to the nursery. They'd ask if they needed a card or something and wouldn't understand until later why I giggled as I told them no card was necessary. "Believe

me, you'll know which one's Brett when you get there!"
"But how will we know which one is Brett? All little
babies look alike." "You'll know," I chuckled, "Just look
for the Angel."

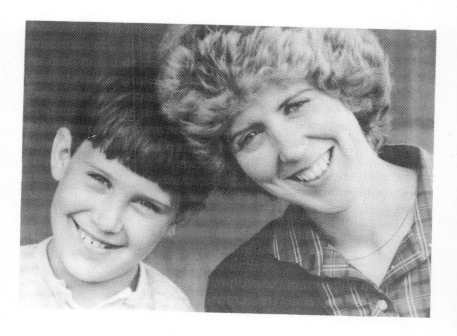

Brett and Patti

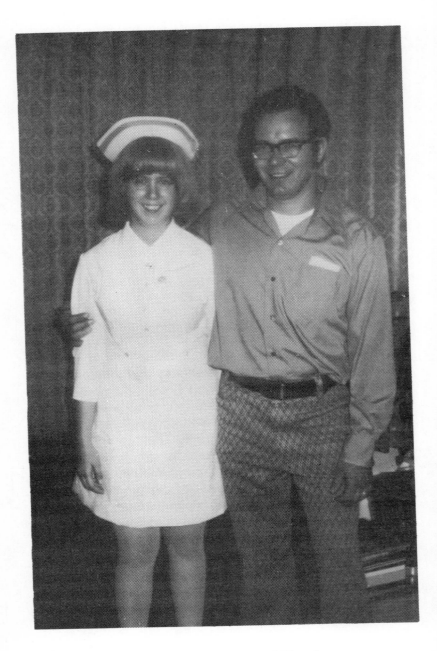

Patti, the nurse and Frank

7

Am I Crazy?

Brett entered the world a holy terror. His crying didn't seem to stop for the first few months of his life on earth. Just when Frank and I thought perhaps that he had some sort of a problem, he changed overnight into a cute, cuddly and for the most part, a quiet precious little boy.

I felt truly blessed by God. I had a good husband whom God had given me in answer to a childhood prayer. My hard-working mate had provided me with a beautiful mobile home with new furnishings at the start of our marriage. And, together we had produced a lovely little baby boy, blessed of God with good health as he entered into to this mixed-up world. Yes, I, Patti Besyk, was really blessed. It was on a Sunday afternoon in the late fall, perhaps September or October, that I was reflecting on these blessings and how great God had been to my little family.

Brett had just been baptised by Pastor Clark and we had returned to Mom and Dad's to celebrate and have dinner. It wasn't that the young Besyk family was materially rich, but I was reflecting on those things that can not be bought at any price. I was meditating on the verses found in Isaiah 55:1-3, "Ho, every one that thirsteth, come ye to the water, and he that hath no money: come ye, buy, and eat; yea, come, buy wine and milk without money and without price. Wherefore do ye spend money for that which is not bread? and your labour for that which satisfieth not? Harken diligently unto me, and eat ye that which is good, and let your should delight itself in fatness. Incline you ear, and come unto me: hear, and your soul shall live; ..." I knew that what really counted in life...the things money could not buy. Aside from Frank, Brett, our new home and furnishings, I had also been blessed with two sets of beautiful parents. Frank's Mom and Dad, in different ways were just as loving and caring as my folks. Though I was shortly beyond the horizon of adulthood myself, I felt my dreams and prayers had all already been answered. My life was roses and blue skies on this lovely fall day. Nothing could possibly change that. It was on that Sunday afternoon at the folk's house that I began to face the fact the roses were wilting and all was not completely well. I bent down to tie little Brett's shoes and things went dark briefly; then the room began to spin like a circus merry-go-round. Had it not happened many times before, I would have simply thought the blood had rushed to my head, or that I got up too quickly. I was proud of being the tomboy outdoor type, and didn't want my family and young groom to know that something was changing inside my body. In my own mind, I knew that I was a strong-willed independent person who could handle anything, and wasn't about to start letting little things get me down at this point in my young life. Maybe my pride hammpered me at this point too, because I didn't want others to begin thinking of me as a hypochondriac! Or, perhaps, I really didn't want to think of myself as one!

It was on that fall Sunday afternoon that I knew something was wrong, really wrong. Something that I knew was only going to get worse. My pride and fears kept me from sharing my sickness with Mom and Dad, let alone with Frank. The dizzy spells became more frequent. Then I began to notice signs that I was losing some of my motor (muscle reflex) control. There would be times when I would be warming a bottle for Brett and would grab the bottle from the boiling water and though I knew it was hot and could feel it burning me, I could not let go of it.

Maybe it was partly because I refused to discuss these fears with anybody that my temperment wick began to burn much shorter, real short! Little things which never used to bother me began to nearly drive me crazy. Months had now passed and little Brett, at 9 months, was beyond the crawling stages and was just starting to discover the independence of walking. As he went from his knees to his feet, Brett discovered a whole new world of curiousities. He was instantly into everything and I began fearing my inability to cope with his natural growth process. I should have been thankful for the healthy progress of my little boy, but my internal turmoil caused rage and bitterness instead of thanksgiving. Still I refused to let down my pride and discuss this with my husband Frank, my mother, my father, or my doctor.

Pride can sometimes become as destructive as any personal problem, and I had a lot of pride and a bunch of unknown fears. I was actually ashamed that something was happening within me that was beyond my control. I was always in control! I also began to fear my resentment of Brett. He was a healthy, happy little boy who was beginning to get into everything, and sometimes I felt like I wanted to spank him, if for no other reason than I felt like it. Then I would catch myself and think, "Am I going to become a child abuser? Am I going crazy? Am I going to go off the handle and hurt Brett? What am I going to do?" Little Brett would be in a kitchen cabinet one minute and under the table the next. In his tiny curious mind, every new moment was an undiscovered adventure. How could he understand why his mother was screaming at him all the time. God help me, even I did not understand why!

"No, I am not going to a doctor." I wrestled with myself. "I can take care of myself. Nobody had to do anything for me." When a Christian, or anybody else for that matter, has a real problem, it is sometimes easier to play ostrich, than to face and deal with the problem. Quite often, when you are a Christian, the problem becomes more compound, because to admit you have a problem, or to dare to seek medical or psychological help can, in the mind, indicate a lack of faith. In my case then, it probably had less to do with faith, than it did with the monumental stumbling block in a meaningfull faith-walk pride. "No," I rationalized, "I am not going to turn into a belly-aching crybaby!"

I was behind the wheel of our car running an errand locally. The day was no different than any other. I am a good driver and the trip was routine. I approached the intersection as the light turned from amber to red. There was pleanty of time to stop. I saw the light change and my brain responded routinely, but my foot did not. It remained on the gas pedal, and my car sped through the traffic light. Thank God there was no intersecting traffic or I might have beem killed! My mind was alert and gave commands to my feet, but there was no response. Once I was able to regain muscle control and bring the car to a complete halt and stop shaking, I knew that I must face my unknown enemy.

In the months since my initial, seemingly innocent, blackouts and dizzy spells, I began experiencing more frequent losses of motor control. I would stumble or fall for no apparent reason. There were times when it seemed as though there was a tight band encasing my chest, and my heart would race almost out of control. After the potential collision in my car, I knew I had to confide in my loved ones, and consult medical help. These things seemed to depart as quickly as they befell me though, and when I consulted my doctor nothing seemed to be wrong. However, my doctor wanted to put me in the hospital for a series of tests. All tests came back negative, which meant, from a medical standpoint, there was nothing wrong with me.

Since nothing showed up on any of the tests, the doctors agreed that I must be suffering from a nervous condition. I had pride, but I was never one to let my nerves run my life. The doctors must know more than I do, so I accepted that it might be nerves, and began taking the prescribed pills.

Once home again, I was groggy and sleepy all the time, and still experiencing the dizziness, blackouts, tightness and rapid heartbeats. The war within my mind was raging. I became more and more convinced that I was, in fact, going crazy! After all, if the doctors couldn't find anything medically wrong with me, then the problem must be emotional.

The situation did not improve. I began to experience a blurriness of vision. I did have glasses for distance, but I so seldom had to wear them that most people didn't know I even wore glasses. One minute I could see clearly and, in an instant, everything, even close up, was a blur. I made an appointment to have my vision checked. After the examination, the eye doctor told me that my problem was not with my eyes, and urged me to consult my family doctor again.

It was no longer the nerve pills which were draining me of my strength. I became weaker and weaker. I didn't even have the ambition or strength, or desire, to take care of Brett or Frank. Poor Frank ended up assuming more and more of the daily responsibility of looking after Brett. And I knew Frank resented it. Maybe the resentment was a display of his pride. Here was his wife, his buddy, who did everything with him, all-of-a-sudden just lying around the house day and night.

I was getting worse and knew it. I tried to be my own doctor, taking mega-doses of vitamins and reading every article I could find on anything which might relate to my undefined situation. Yes, I did return to the doctors, but the doctors continued to find nothing in their tests.

Up to this point, my stubborn pride had kept me from confiding in Mom and Dad. There came a day when I unwillingly confided in them. I was at their house doing some seeding in the back yard, something I had done hundreds of times before. But this time was different. One minute I was bending down, and the next I heard myself scream out for help before everything went dark. Dad found me unconscious in the dirt. He wanted to call an ambulance, but I pleaded with him, "Don't do that Dad, I'm fine, I'll be all right." Dad honored my wish and an ambulance was not summoned. In spite of my stubbornness, the cloud hovering over my life did not evaporate. It only grew darker. Not long after my fainting spell, I had to call out to Dad again. It was a Sunday morning; I was not feeling well so I stayed home with Brett while Frank and Mom attended church together. Dad has black-lung disease and had his ups-and-downs too. That particular Sunday morning, he was not up to going to church.

After Frank left, I began to feel something I had not experienced before. I simply felt like I was going to die. My fear may not have been so much for me as for little Brett. "Dad, come over here. Something is wrong," I breathed into the phone. The distance between the two homes was only about a city block, so Dad arrived almost instantaneously. He immediately called the hospital emergency room. After explaining to the doctor on duty that I was on nerve medication, Dad was instructed to double the medication. If it was a mistake on the part of the doctor, I know it was an honest mistake. Dad did as instructed. After that, the situation grew worse. I slipped in and out of consciousness, and my fingernails began to turn blue.

Dad frantically called the emergency room again and, after explaining my condition to the doctor, was instructed to call an ambulance immediately and get me down to the hospital. The doctor who had instructed him to get me to the hospital went off duty before I arrived, but had left instructions to give me some vallium, that I had a nervous condition. Drugs on top of drugs! I was sent home and became less and less able to function as a wife, mother or human being.

Mom was now watching Brett more and more. Mom really loved her troubled daughter and grandson and related to me the new and exciting things Brett did in any given day, but I cared less and less. My mind and instincts were so fogged by that point. It bothered me that I didn't even care, that I didn't care!

Kathy was always my very best friend and she is to this day, but at this point in Frank and my lives, God managed to bring two other people into our lives, Jerry and Beth. Frank and Jerry became acquainted through a mutual infatuation with snowmobiling. Soon Frank and Jerry were the best of friends. Frank raced and Jerry was the mechanic. As a result of that Beth and I were thrown together as snowmobile widows, in that neither of us enjoyed the racing part of the outdoor sport. We did however, enjoy the sport. As a result we became friends, good friends.

Beth was an RN, Registered Nurse. As we became friends and I related my experiences to Beth, her RN instinct sparked Beth's professional ire! Maybe she was seeing things that my doctors had missed, or maybe she had become too emotionally attached to me to be professionally objective. "There's a doctor I'd like you to see," Beth said to me. I agreed to an appointment. For whatever reason, this was the first doctor who conducted a simple test, taking my blood pressure while I was lying down and then immediately when I stood up. Why the others didn't do this, I don't know, but this doctor must have seen something in the comparison, whether or not he initially understood what he was seeing. Most important to me was the fact that this doctor didn't think I was whacko or a hypochondriac. He said to me, "Patti, something more is wrong. We have to find out. We just can't keep letting it go. If it's something we can control, then we've got to catch it now and not let it go on." For me, that was a great relief, to have a doctor climb inside my emotional shell and tell me I was not crazy.

This doctor was convinced that there was more to my problem than had been diagnosed by other doctors to this point. That was really reasurring to me. Hospital rooms and the routine were becoming all too familiar to me. It was no longer a day or two for tests, but a week or two, or a month! I became used to being shuffled from room to room, and ward to ward, Foreign gadgets strapped or inserted into my body became more and more common. It's a weird, and degrading, situation to be so wired up that a faceless, nameless person down the hall can tell, from a television monitor, when you even burp!

The regimented routine of a hospital environment becomes so mundane to the patient that even the bland meal becomes an event, three times a day! I faded in and out of reality more and more. Even though, in my spasms with reality, I knew that Mom was caring for Brett and Frank was going home to an empty place nightly. I simply didn't care. Brett was too young to be allowed into my room, so Frank would bring him to the hospital and just stand with him on the sidewalk below my room so that the little guy could see his mommy, and his mommy could wave to him if she even cared at that point. And, at that point I did not care. They were simply a man with a cute little boy waving in my direction. There were no emotional ties on my part at that point.

An internist from another hospital visited me. He was interested in my case and wanted to treat me, but I would have to transfer to Windber Hospital. It was a little closer to Mom and Dad's, but further from where Frank worked. His job was in Johnstown, not far from Memorial Hospital, so Frank could stop in and visit me every evening on his way home from work. Now that I was being transferred to the hospital in Windber, it meant Frank would be running himself ragged between home, work and the hospital. The three sites formed a near perfect triangle for Frank instead of a straight line, as before.

I was becoming less and less concerned with those who loved me, and more wrapped up in me, Patti Besyk. When I would call Mom, I didn't want to hear about what, or how, Brett was doing, or how they were doing, or how Frank was doing. I wanted Mom to ask how I was doing! It hurt Mom that I was losing hold of my love for all of them, but she never said anything.

In my self-centered state of mind, I didn't care about anybody but Patti. And I was glad that there was something wrong with me. That is not to say that I was glad to have, as yet, an undiagnosed illness, but glad, or relieved, that maybe the doctors would finally begin to get at the root of my problem.

Frank had visited me at the Johnstown hospital daily like clockwork. On the day I was transferred to Windber, Frank didn't come for hours. Though I didn't really appreciate his visits at Memorial, my mind was so twisted then, after a few hours in my new room at Windber, I resented the fact that he hadn't shown up yet. How dare him! A nurse about then entered my room and handed me a pill and said, "Please take this, Patti." "What is it for?" I demanded. The nurse tried to encourage me to take it, but I flatly refused. It was just a tranquilizer. The nurse knew something I didn't.

After what seemed like hours, Frank and Mom walked into my hospital room. My internal rage was squelched when I looked at their somber faces. I knew in a instant that something had happened. Something was wrong. Frank stood there and stared at me and finally mumbled, "Patti, honey, my Mother is dead. She died." I couldn't believe what I was hearing and said, "Frank, your Mother is what?" "She is dead," he slowly repeated himself. "So that is the reason the nurse had encouraged me to take the tranquilizer," I said. The ward nurse had been alerted that the mother of the husband of their newest patient had died just a few hours before, and they didn't know how I would react, so they wanted to sedate me.

What the nurses didn't know was, at that point in my illness, I could have cared less, about anybody or anything. Though Frank's parents had been very good to us. I felt nothing! In my present frazzled emotional state when I didn't even care about my husband, little Brett or anybody else, why would anyone think I would weep over the loss of my Mother-in-law? My emotional mind was almost totally gone and nobody seem to understand. Not even me. Frank didn't cry, Mom didn't cry, nor did I. None of us were from an emotional background to start with. It didn't mean that we were cold or heartless or uncaring people, though I was at this point, it simply meant we didn't know how to cry. A lot of people are that way, so they cry on the inside while their eyes remain dry. As for me, I did feel somewhat bad for Frank, but that was the extent of my remorse. "What dreadful illness is causing me to be this way?" I thought.

Most of Frank's relatives lived in other parts of the country, so many traveled long distances to attend the funeral and needed places to stay. Mom and Dad ended up making up all kinds of sleeping accommodations for the strangers. Others stayed at our place with Frank. "Probably on dirty sheets," I thought later.

"How did she die?" I quizzed Frank. Frank didn't answer me and quickly turned the conversation to something else. He was very uneasy and after a few minutes said he had to leave. Frank's mother had been sick and the doctors had been pumping all kinds of medicine into her. She had little brown pill bottles everywhere and I am certain that she didn't even know why she was taking most of the stuff. This always bothered me and I was concerned about all of the medications various doctors were now prescribing for me. It was my body, and I didn't want to be any doctor's guinea pig!

"How did she die?" I asked my friend Beth on the phone. After Frank had excused himself so abruptly, I had immediately called Beth. "Look, Beth, I want to know what is going on. I want to know the truth. I know you didn't want to break the news to me and tell me she died, but now I want to know how she died." There was a long pause. Finally Beth said, "Patti, she took her own life." It confirmed what I had suspected, and nobody would ever convince me that the combination of medications prescribed by various doctors didn't eventually cause a chemical reaction in her system which was an emotional time bomb that eventually exploded! "Patti, please don't let anyone know that I have told you. You are my best friend and you asked me, so I told you. Please promise me you won't tell anyone," Beth asked. Beth and Jerry rented from Frank's parents, and their house was right next door. When Frank's father found that his wife was dead, he ran next door to get them. He was probably clinging to the hope that it was not too late, but it was.

It was ironic that Frank's mother was buried on my birthday. It was not, needless to say, a happy one. There I was, confined to my hospital room, feeling like a prisoner while my husband attended his mother's funeral. That was the only time that I wept. It was not for my deceased Mother-in-law, but for my husband, going through this grief without me at his side. I came out of my self-centered shell briefly, and cried for my poor husband.

After the funeral Frank came to visit me. He and Mom had gotten permission to bring Brett into my room. In Frank's grief, he still remembered that it was my birthday. They brought a cake and a tennis racquet, ball and even a hat. I had always wanted to learn tennis, so they bought me the tools to learn. In my mind, and theirs too, whatever was wrong with me would not last long, so I would soon get out of the hospital and learn to play tennis! Maybe I was just clinging to hope at that point. After a forced birthday party, they all left. I was tired and wanted to go to sleep and forget...forget.

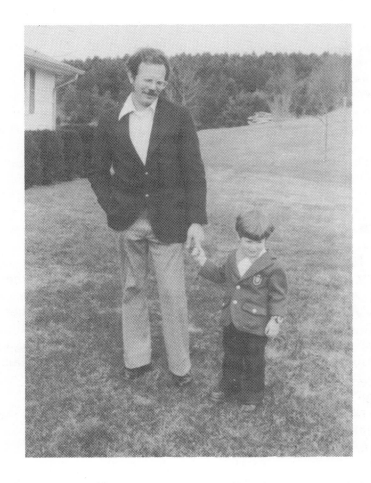

Frank and Brett, waiting alone

8

You Have Multiple Sclerosis

When you are admitted to the hospital for tests, you quickly start feeling like a human guinea pig. Even though the doctors are truly searching for the problem, you can quickly develop the helpless feeling that they don't know any more about what's wrong with you than you do! I had so many blood tests on a regular basis that I began to feel like a pin cushion. When science and medicine are seeking a solution, they often have to play the odds by process of elimination. Based on the information they have as a result of tests, they resort to trying this or that medicine. If it helps to improve the condition, they can assume they're on the right track. Based on my symptoms and the results of my tests, they would prescribe a new medication. Often it would help, temporarily, but the same symptoms would soon reoccur.

The latest medication seemed promising so, after a month or so in the Windber hospital, I was released. It was springtime and I took notice of the beauty of the season change like never before.

I was truly thankful that I was out of the hospital,

back at home, and that the long ordeal was over. The family was back together again and life was nice once more.

The interlude, though brief, was beautiful while it lasted. Maybe a few relatively normal months passed. There were minor dizzy spells, but I fooled myself into believing that they were normal. Then the blackouts returned and increased along with a new experience, seizures. The latest medication was no longer helping at all. One day Mom and I went to the doctor for a routine exam. As I was paying the bill, I said to Mom, "It's happening!"

Mom didn't know what I meant until I collapsed! I could always tell when "it" was going to happen. Everything would start to have a kind of rosey, red glow around it. Then I would see a sort-of halo, then darkness. One minute I was paying the bill at the doctor's office, and the next minute I was in an ambulance en route to the hospital again. My doctor knew there was something wrong, but didn't know what. I was placed in Intensive Care. I was in Intensive Care on the critical list, but nobody, including the doctors, knew why.

Whatever it was, my condition would leave as quickly as it arrived. In short order, I was transferred from Intensive Care to a regular intermediate ward. Believe it or not, a really good and alert doctor or nurse is encouraged by patient complaining! It is a sign of increasing wellness! A really sick patient may complain about pain or discomfort, but one en route to recovery will begin to complain about the lousy food or the bad TV reception or whatever. Well, the doctors and nurses were encouraged when I began to gripe about these very things! Their encouragement was short-lived.

Yes, the TV reception was not the best, and the food could be resented by anybody, especially when you consider what you're paying for food which is void of any real flavor. I began complaining about things which the doctors knew went beyond healthy griping. But the doctors couldn't really find anything wrong, so they sent me home again.

Once again in familiar surroundings, I tried to convince myself that the worst was over. My body would not confirm that wish. My legs began to do funny things. They didn't really hurt, but they began to co-operate less and less with what my mind told them to do. Though I was not given to alcohol consumption, I had begun to feel drunk when even walking around the house. I had experienced the glow of a taste of wine at my wedding reception so I thought I knew what it felt like. Now I sometimes experienced the "buzz" without the consumption! Something was wrong! I was even tripping and stumbling on flat surfaces within my own home.

The medical tests continued. I was now losing not only physical motor co-ordination with my legs, but also with my bladder. My bladder would no longer fully empty as it should. It seemed as though my nerves, or responses, were becoming more deadened or independent.

The all-too-familiar surroundings of a hospital room became home for me again. I was in my home one minute, and in the hospital bed the next. My legs, acting independently of my mind, apparently just gave out! I fell. I broke not only my elbow, but a few ribs too! It was a total blackout and I awoke in a hospital room! When I regained consciousness, my arm was in a cast and my chest was wrapped in tape.

Pastor Clark was there. He always was there! And he always looked on the bright side of a situation, but when your arm is in a cast, your ribs are encased in tape, and you are in pain, it's hard to believe that God really loves you. Many evangelists use the slogan, "God loves you." But, when you are in pain, it is sometimes hard to believe it!

This time, the doctors must have known that something was going on inside me that they could not diagnose. There was no time left to allow any personal medical ego trips infringe on my right to become well. Thus, I was transferred to West Penn Hospital in Pittsburgh, eons away from my familiar surroundings.

In Johnstown Memorial or the hospital in Windber, I was still in familiar territory. But Pittsburgh was so far away. No longer could Mom or Frank pop in nightly. The phone bill grew rapidly. I was afraid and alone. When I called home, I wanted to know that I was wanted, missed, and cared about. I needed to be needed, and resented it when Mom or Frank would conversationally begin to tell me about what was going on on the home front. From their standpoint, they were saying things they thought I wanted to know about. From my standpoint, I needed to have their conversation center around me.

The tests continued, but the doctors discovered nothing. I was removed from some of the medications, but the root problem was not diagnosed, and I was sent home.

It was the Christmas season when I was released from the Pittsburgh hospital. Our close friends were so special, along with women from the church. I was released from the Pittsburgh hospital the week before Christmas and returned to find that people, out of love, had cleaned my home, baked holiday goodies and wrapped gifts. They had displayed what true Christian love is all about without any demand for personal recognition. It was difficult for me to grasp such unconditional caring!

The holiday season passed, but my condition continued. My test results from Pittsburgh were sent to Dr. Caroff. He had become my local hope. "Did you hear from the doctor out of Pittsburgh?" I asked on my first visit after the holidays. "Yes, I have. Patti, have you ever heard of Multiple Sclerosis?", he asked. "Yes", I responded, but my mind was saying, "No way will I have it. I don't have it and I won't have it, because I don't have time for it." After months of testing, my mind was fighting facing reality. I knew enough about MS to know that it eventually could totally cripple and disable you. I would not end up in a wheel chair.

"Is there a cure for it?", I finally heard myself ask the

doctor. His one word answer was, "No." The doctors can tell you that science is on the edge of a cure, but when you are the diagnosed person involved, it is hard to buy their encouragement! Multiple Sclerosis has varying degrees. There are mild cases, where the person can lead a relatively normal life, and then there are the extreme cases where the person becomes totally dependent on others to care for him or her. I feared the latter.

"I have MS." I shared with Frank once I was able to go home again. "What's that?" Frank rightfully asked innocently. Though he was a man of the world in my eyes, Frank was naive about such medical things. He truly wanted to know what our mutual future held. We went over to Jerry and Beth's place. Because she was an RN, Beth had several medical books. We researched Multiple Sclerosis. At that point, I determined that I had the mild case and not the totally helpless advanced stages of MS. Even though I had determined that I had the mild MS condition, my body would not confirm my determination. I began limping more. My legs didn't hurt, but there was simply less co-ordination.

Tests continued, diagnoses continued, and the regular visits to the Pittsburgh hospital continued. After a year in and out of the Pittsburgh hospital, all I had to show for the multi-efforts was a set of very basic wooden crutches. They would help me walk instead of stumble around the house. I had no real prolonged stays in the hospital, but was given the tools I needed to stumble through the routine of basic life in familiar surroundings.

Things went downhill from that point. My particular type of MS was apparently the one which advanced rapidly. There was no real remission, though there were days when I would feel perfectly fine. There was a false hope each time I went through a battery of tests and was sent home. Anything was better than having to stay in the hospital, but the frequency of my stays increased.

In my case, it may have been a multiple physical problem. Many of my symptoms were not common to MS patients. The blackouts and the eventual internal bleeding were not symptoms common to the MS sufferer.

After my transfer, and initial release, from the pittsburgh hospital, I was in and out of the hospital nearly monthly for the next three years. The medications continued. On my later stays in the Pittsburgh hospital, I was put on steroids which eventually caused gastric bleeding. This had nothing to do directly with MS, but it my case, was the stressful result of MS.

The more frequent stays in the hospital were emotionally draining me. They were probably also emotionally draining Frank, Mom, and Dad. They proved their love and loyalty in countless ways. Not only when I was afraid and alone in some strange hospital room, but also, more importantly, when I was at home. In those times, maybe, they coddled me too much for my emotional good. They were living their love for me daily even when, in the depths of my self-centeredness, I wasn't always a willing recipient.

I had always feared becoming a cripple or dependent on others. I was thankful that once I had to begin using crutches, Frank never made me feel like a cripple. When I was feeling up to it, we even took motorcycle rides together. Frank would simply strap my crutches, or crunches as Brett called them, on the safety bar, and off we'd go just like old times.

How great it was to be free from the prison walls of the hospital. Even having to use crutches was a small price to pay for my freedom. But that freedom was short lived. I began experiencing an upset stomach on a regular basis. Then I began vomiting, and finally, began spitting up blood. The doors were slammed shut on my temporary freedom as I was, once again, admitted into the hospital.

I was given shots of demerol to control the pain. "Boy, these shots could make a drug addict out of you in a big hurry." I told my doctor. "I can see why people like them." They'd give me a shot and, whew, I was on cloud nine. I could care less what happened in the world. The internal bleeding was brought under control and I was sent home once again.

My blackouts increased in frequency. The specialists explained to me, in laymen's terms, that when you stand up, your nerves automatically send impulses to your veins to constrict so that gravity wouldn't drain the blood from the brain too quickly. In my case, the impulses weren't reaching the veins, so when I would stand up too quickly, my brain would instantly be drained of blood, causing the blackouts. One minute I'd be sitting or bending over and the next instant I'd get light headed and everything would go black. Then I would awaken on the couch where Frank, Dad, or Mom had moved me from where I had fallen and the ambulance would already be there. Sirens wailing and it was back to the hospital. The routine was becoming all too familiar for all of us. For me, it was becoming a nightmare! A living hell!

The seizures could no longer be controlled. It was back to Johnstown Memorial. Once again, I was placed in Intensive Care. I was in and out of consciousness. "I don't understand it," the doctor told Dad. "We have given her enough medicine to knock down a horse and still we can't calm the seizures." Every time I would have a seizure, it was so violent that I would literally burn up over 600 calories! My weight decreased rapidly, as seizure followed seizure.

The combination of grand mals and MS was like a molitov cocktail exploding inside of me. It was starting to take its toll on the nerve points to my brain. The fine line between reality and nightmare ceased to be. It all blended together into a minute by minute nightmare. I was in and out of comas. I could no longer distinguish between what was real and what seemed real. The seizures, medication, and MS all worked as a team to cause mental suicide at that point.

"The nurses had a party last night," I told Mom. "I could have died and they wouldn't have known. They were dancing in the halls and everything." Of course, there was no party except in my hallucinations.

Frank, Mom, Dad, they all tried to put on a happy face for their loved one, but how it ripped them apart inside each time they visited their helpless trooper. And I was a trooper. I was losing the battle, and how each of them sobbed internally as they smiled outwardly for my sake.

"Don't let them take me." I would sob. The fear was very real in my eyes. "Who?" Mom gently prodded, clutching my hand as she sat beside my bed. "Them! The helicopter. They are going to take me!" I yelled as I pointed to the window of my hospital room. My room at Memorial overlooked the parking lot. The tall light poles which illuminated the lot extended to eye level with my window. What I saw as I lay in my bed at night was the tops of the umbrella shaped lamp posts. What my mind saw was helicopters hovering outside my window waiting to snatch me away. Or maybe they were aliens in foreign spacecraft. There was no difference in my mind at that point. I was scared to death of a threat which my mind had produced. Whether real or imagined, fear can be the real enemy. Franklin D. Roosevelt once said, "We have nothing to fear, but fear itself." The medical profession might disagree with F.D.R'S analysis of mankind's deepest problem, but he may have been more right than wrong.

My complications mounted. Not only were the effects of MS draining life from my young body, but my weight loss had reached the critical level. In my hospital bed, I looked like a skeleton covered by a sheet. The team of doctors could not allow me to lose any more weight. An incision was made at my collar bone and a tube was inserted. The incision was stitched around the tube. The tube apparently served a dual purpose. Not only did it force nourishment into my rapidly deteriorating body, but it also allowed the doctors and nurses to constantly monitor my blood pressure right in my heart.

Had my mind been rational, I would have asked God, "Why?" But Frank, Mom, Dad, and others must have asked that question many times. They went to church. They were ethical and moral people. Their faith and religion was not something which any of them took superficially. "Why, God?" The answer did not come from the heavens as they watched my condition worsen.

My ability to breathe declined. It was no longer a matter of hooking me up to oxygen. I now needed a respirator to force me to breathe. It would force air into my lungs. I was not permitted off the respirator unless someone else was in the room with me. When Dad would come to visit me, it would tear him apart inside to have to say, "Patti, breathe." Without the machine, my lungs would no longer respond to the brain's automatic signal instructing me to breathe.

Two weeks of my life have been snuffed from my memory. I have no recollection of what went on. I was in Intensive Care, not being able to breathe on my own, and then I awoke one day in another room, on another floor. I was feeling friskier than I had in ages. It wasn't that I was feeling good, but for the first time in quite awhile, I was simply feeling.

"I feel like a Mac truck ran over me." I complained to my doctor. "No wonder," he reassured me, "with all the seizures you had, it's no wonder you ache all over." This was the same doctor, a Christian, who told my folks, "It's in God's hands. If she's going to live, it's in His hands now. We've done all we can do for her." The doctor's compassionate, faith-filled honesty ripped away at their hearts. Yet they knew they had to remain strong for my sake and strong they remained.

Hospital! Home! Hospital! Home! It became such an emotional Ping-Pong game for all of us. "Let her do anything she can." The doctor advised as I was about to be released from the hospital again. He probably didn't want me to feel like an invalid any sooner than necessary.

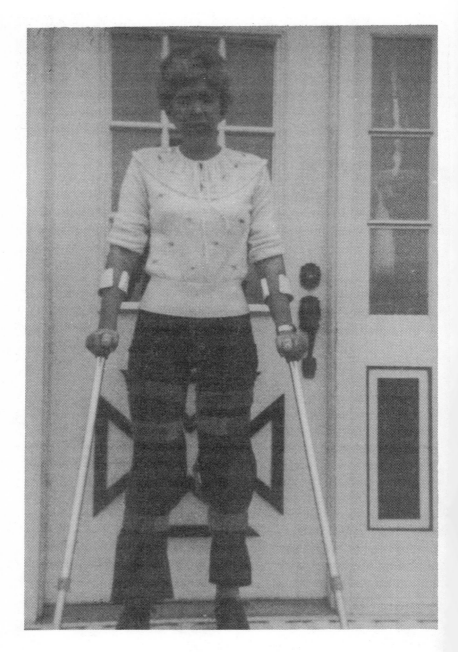

"Braced" for a walk

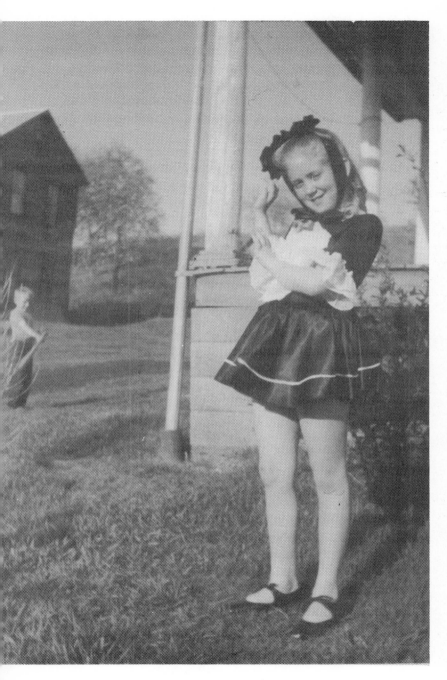

My Sears' dancing outfit

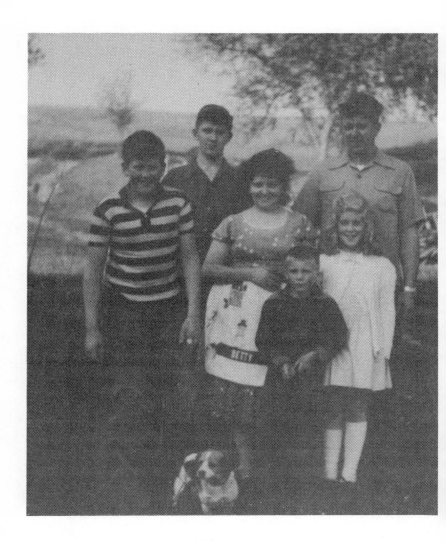

My Family

9

Moments To Live

At home, it was hard for me to try even the simple things. I was now on crutches all the time. Even trying to hang one of Frank's shirts on a hanger was an ordeal. It was even more of an ordeal for Mom, who sat by watching as she fought the urge to say, "Here, Patti, let me do that for you." Though they were all crying inside, they knew that each of them had to let me try to do everything I could on my own. It was important for me to maintain some feeling of independence for as long as I could.

Pastor Clark was always faithful to visit me, whether in my hospital room or at home. His visits were becoming more and more of an irritant to me. This dear person would pray for me and all the time my resentment grew. "Hey, you've been praying for me for two years now, since the very first," I thought, "and I've just gotten worse. What kind of wool are you trying to pull over my eyes? Nothing's happened, and nothing's going to happen." There were those good Christians who would question my lack of faith, but those same people have never walked in my shoes or with my crutches.

Maybe they should thank God that they never have.

It may not have been actual remission, but things temporarily seemed to settle on an even keel. I wasn't getting better, but neither was I getting worse. It was a temporary plateau that, at that point, I could have been content to live on for the rest of my life. Then one day I fell off the end of the plateau and ended up back in the hospital. This time, the problem was bursitis in my shoulders. Crutches are only meant for temporary use, perhaps six weeks. I had been on them for nearly a year and my shoulders were now rebelling.

The medication was apparently prescribed to block off, or deaden, the irritated nerves in my shoulders. They probably used novocaine. Whatever it was, my system rebelled violently and I was placed in Intensive Care again. The doctors had no way of knowing that I was allergic to novocaine. My veins collapsed after the initial injection. They had to get me on I.V., but couldn't find a vein. The passage of time was critical. There wasn't a minute to lose. The doctors had to cut directly into my arms simply in hopes of finding a vein. After that, they began inserting I.V. needles into my legs, my feet, anywhere they could locate a vein which might serve the purpose.

Eventually my condition stabilized so I was moved to an intermediate care room once again. My weight continued to dwindle, so the team of doctors decided to try something new on me. It seemed to me they were always trying something new, but at that point, what did they have to lose? The latest experiment was a spaghetti tube. It looked exactly like a strand of spaghetti and was threaded up my nose and down my throat. The exposed end was connected to an I.V. bag which would, one drop at a time, force nourishment into my stomach.

I was in pain most of the time and the severity of my discomfort increased. Finally, I was given pain shots. The shots gave temporary relief, but after awhile, I feared that I was becoming a junkie. I began staring at my watch to see when I would receive the next injection. Soon I was ringing my buzzer demanding another pain shot, though it may only have been twenty or thirty minutes since the last injection. At that point, I know I could probably have been classified as a drug addict.

While in Memorial Hospital, I met Dr. Smith, the first female doctor to counsel me. Dr. Smith had done her internship at St. Francis Hospital, a Catholic hospital in Pittsburgh, which specializes in rehabilitation. She felt that they could help me, but it would involve my being transferred to the Pittsburgh facility. Frank, Mom, Dad, and I all agreed. So once again, I found myself in strange surroundings, but strangely different from the other hospitals in which I had been.

At St. Francis, they encouraged an independent attitude. They gently forced their residents to function on their own so that they would not feel like invalids. Developing that particular attitude was important in the success of any future rehabilitation attempts. You also wore street clothes rather than those humiliating hospital gowns which must have been designed to fit everybody, and yet seemed to fit nobody right.

My first morning at St. Francis, an attendant entered my room and asked me what I wanted to wear that day from the selection of street clothing I had brought. Once I had responded, the woman removed the garments from the closet, placed them on the bed, and said, "OK, here they are. I'll be back shortly. Get yourself ready." At this stage of my multiple diseases and disorders, I had lost almost all of my motor functions. My legs and arms just wouldn't respond when my mind commanded them to. Perhaps a half hour later the nurse returned and I had barely even begun to dress myself.

The St. Francis rehabilitation program strived to de-emphasize a traditional hospital atmosphere in favor of a more informal setting. Not only did patients wear street clothes, but they also ate together in a dining room. Unless a patient was bedridden, there was no breakfast in bed. I was just not prepared for this sudden change in my routine. More than anything, I wanted the security of my pain shots. This security, and the resulting tranquility, had been instantly withheld from me and my system rebelled, quickly, and violently. I was suddenly going through emotional and physical drug withdrawal!

Though I was one of St. Francis' newer patients, I was not one of their more routine cases. I was received as a rehab patient. For some reason, my medical records did not immediately accompany me to St. Francis, so the nurses and doctors may not have been familiar enough with my complex case. Maybe nobody, whether at Memorial or at St. Francis, could have realized the chemical dependency my body had developed for the pain shots, but I knew. When my system was instantly robbed of this euphoria, it fought back. Though I hadn't experienced a seizure in quite a while, I went into seizures again. The staff at St. Francis was caught totally off guard.

Had it not been for a nameless nurse, my life would have ended at St. Francis. Alone in my room, I went into a seizure and could not breathe. This particular nurse entered my room and immediately realized the severity of the situation. "She absolutely has to be moved. Something's wrong," the nurse told the physician on duty. Tracking the doctor down and stating her evaluation could only have taken a few minutes away from my bedside, but it was long enough for my system to begin shutting down. When the nurse returned, my heart had stopped. I was not breathing. I was, in fact, dead at that point!

Had the nurse panicked upon returning to the room, my life's story would have ended there, nothing more than a story of trials, courage and defeat. The nurse wasted no time in administering CPR. My system may have been in the process of closing shop, but the initial CPR efforts of this particular nurse forced my body to resentfully begin responding again. I was then immediately wisked to intensive care.

Anybody who has ever sat with a comatose person in a

hospital room may talk to that un-responding person wondering what purpose it serves to talk to someone who apparently doesn't hear those words. Though the patient seems completely unresponsive, never doubt that person's ability to hear and understand your words. Even a person who is nearing death can hear, though his or her body can no longer respond. Even one whose body is preparing to exit this life will hear a simple, "I love you", whispered through tears. There may be no physical indication, but the heart and pulse monitors will always indicate an acknowledgement.

Such was the case with me as I was being rushed to intensive care. Though I could not talk, see, move, or in any other way, respond, I could still hear. As two nurses were wheeling me up to intensive care on the gurney, I could hear their conversation. Something about a rock concert in Pittsburgh and the whole rock-drug scene. As they talked, I imagined the two nurses looking down at my body thinking that she was one of these freaked-out, overdosed druggies. How could these nurses know that I was not a doper, though I was apparently dependent on drugs at this point. How could they know that I was not some "hippie" throwing my life away on drugs and booze? How could they know that I could hear every word they were saying as they wheeled my un-responsive body to intensive care?

The Intensive Care Unit at St. Francis did not involve individual rooms as it had at Memorial. I was put in a ward with several other patients. My body did not give any indication of being alert, but I remember the sounds of my stay in St. Francis' intensive care. My ears became sightless eyes. I could hear and sense the presence of another person. Even the quiet rustle of a skirt or nylon jacket. They all had different and distinct characteristics which go totally unnoticed when the eyes and other senses are functioning. In my dark comatose world, even when a word was not spoken, the sound of another person's breathing, or the rustling of their clothing was so reassuring, for I knew somebody else was with me, and cared enough to be there.

In intensive care, I soon regained consciousness. The initial life and death battle was over, but my body cried out for the drugs it had come to depend on. They had to treat me as a common drug addict, which I was. I was, at times, a wild person. Leather bindings had to be employed to restrict my arms and legs. The body of one going through drug or alcohol withdrawal can develop superhuman spurts of strength. I was no different. My surges of strength would sometimes break the leather restraints.

Just as I saw hovering helicopters outside my room at Memorial, my mind would now see snakes and spiders crawling all over my cubicle at St. Francis. In my mind, what I saw was real. I screamed and cried and fought to free myself from the leather restraints. I soon developed a craftiness. Once I regained consciousness, I learned to play on the sympathy of Frank, the folks or anybody else who visited me. "Oh, these straps hurt me so much," I would whine, "please loosen them a little." They would be temporarily loosened, but when my visitor left, the restraints would always be tightened in spite of my protests.

As my withdrawal symptoms decreased, I graduated from leather to cloth restraints. My craftiness grew. I learned how to make a fist when the nurse would apply the cloth restraint around my arms. Though my body weight at that point had dwindled to, perhaps, 90 pounds, even flexing a small muscle when the restraints are applied can mean freedom when the nurse has left! It became so easy for me to get out of my shackles once the nurse was gone.

The human body going through chemical withdrawal reacts like a dry sponge in search of water. It needs the revitalization which only water or drugs can bring at that point. In my own case, I wanted to die! It would have to be better than what my body was going through. Even hell, in my drug-starved state, would have to be better than what I was experiencing. When you need a "fix", whether food, water, drugs, or booze, you need it now!

As the days passed, my chemical need for drugs decreased, but my emotional need continued to rebel. Who but God knows what happened, or why, at that point in my life. Was it the MS, the need for drugs, the withdrawal from drugs, which seemed to defy any medical attempts to restore me to health? In any case, I reached a point in time where the medical profession could do no more.

My trips into and out of reality continued, even though the snakes and spiders of my mind had exited for the most part. My bouts with delirium tremens continued. One particular night, when I was in and out of consciousness or reality, I could hear, in my physically unresponsive state, the urgency of the nurses outside my room. "She's not going to make it through the night, we'd better call her minister." Though I was physically unresponsive, the eye of my ear could hear what was going on. Papers rustled as the nurses looked for Pastor Clark's number. "Oh no, he lives so far away. He will never be able to get here in time." I knew they were talking about me.

"No", I said in my mind, "I won't die!" Since the nurses didn't think I could last long enough for Pastor Clark to arrive, they summoned the Catholic Priest on duty and he entered my room and administered Last Rites. "No Way", I silently shouted in my mind, "No way am I going to die."

"Oh, her husband is so young," I heard one nurse say to another. "I wonder if he will remarry. I wonder if his new wife will want to adopt his son?" "Hey, I am not dead. Please wait," my mind cried out though my voice was able to say nothing to those hovering over me.

Needless to say I did not die. My condition eventually improved enough to where I was moved from intensive care and back into the regular St. Francis rehabilitation Program. The regime was again dressing yourself, going to therapy, and the cafeteria. You were expected to function within a group environment and not alone. I learned how to operate a wheel chair. I may have wanted to withdraw at that point, but the St. Francis program would not permit your being in your room unless it was to sleep. When you went to your room and hopped into bed, it was time to sleep. Otherwise, there was no reason for being alone in your room or bed! That was the St. Francis brand of therapy.

Maybe out of mutual self-defense, Dan, another patient and I became close comrades. It might have been because we were the two youngest patients in St. Francis' therapy at that time. We were surrounded by amputees, stroke victims and others. And all seemed to be much older than Dan and I. We emotionally needed, and leaned upon each other during that time. How it must have hurt Frank to make the 80-mile trip nightly to be with me, only to hear about Dan .. Dan .. Dan. How could he understand that we were both cripples, both young, both scared, and then, both needing each other. Though it may have hurt him, Frank never said a word.

It was nearing Thanksgiving. "I can get you a pass to go home for Thanksgiving," my counselor said to me. "Frank could come and get you, then bring you back Thanksgiving night." "NO WAY!" I responded. "You send me home and I'll never come back. You will have to beat me over the head with a hammer to get me back." I spent Thanksgiving, and the rest of the holidays, in the hospital. Dan did too. I had arm braces by that time. Dan had a broken back. Others had experienced strokes and other disabilitating encounters. It must have been quite a sight to the outside observer as food flew everywhere in the patients' attempts to guide the holiday meal to their mouths. Often it would end up on their shoulders, their chests or back on the plate from which it came. But there was a silent comradery among us.

My nurses couldn't get over the mail I received. I was never forgotten by my church. There are those who are of the opinion that Lutherans are rather cold, uncaring people, but don't ever tell me that unless you are prepared for a strong and lengthy rebuttal. There was one family in particular, a mother and her two daughters, who saw to it that I got a card and a note every day. Yes, everyday! Each of the three had assigned days of the week to send a card and note, and none ever missed a day!

Others in my small Lutheran congregation, even people I barely knew, sent letters and cards on a regular basis. The church family and my own family were supportive in all ways, cards, notes, letters and regular visits. It is easy to feel very lonely in a hospital environment, but my family and friends did everything humanly possible to let me know constantly that I was loved.

In many ways for me, the time had dragged since I first entered the hospital centuries earlier, but in ways which cut more deeply, it had flown. Little Brett was four years old or so and it pained me to know that Brett and I had been robbed of those very special early years when a mother is the central figure in a toddler's life. Mom had been both grandmother and mother to Brett. She fed him, clothed him, bathed him, sang songs to him, all the things I should have been doing. But Mom never tried to replace me in Brett's life and always kept his young mind alive with his mother's presence, even in her absence.

Going to visit his mommy was a big event in his little life. On one occasion, around the holidays, he wanted a red sweater to wear to see me. He was so proud and looked so cute. Brett was always singing too. He would sing for me at home, and Mom would often write down the lyrics for me. At that time, my emotions teetered between feeling guilt at having not been much a part of Brett's life those first four years, and just not really caring. In a lot of ways, I became used to the hospital routine and my new friends there. It was a different world, but my world, and Brett, Frank, and the rest of them just didn't fit into that world! It was never a case of not loving them, but simply I didn't feel anything toward them at that particular emotional hour of my life.

It would be easy for them to question how I could possibly have grown so cold toward those who really meant something in my life. To question is understandable, but to judge is another matter. They never once judged me. Unless we have walked in another's shoes, or better yet, walked barefoot over the hot coals of their crisis, none has the right to judge. The Bible commands us to do the opposite! Frank, the folks and my friends did just that!

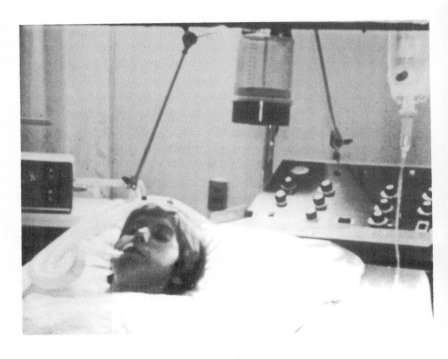

Dying

10

St. Francis Hospital

I became classified as a non-conformist, a trouble-maker by the doctors, nurses and therapists at St. Francis. It wasn't that I was downright nasty, just cantankerous, or more often than not, just plain ornery! My therapists were frustrated with my constant frustration! And frustrated I was. I once threw a shoe at my therapist and screamed, "You know, the problem is I have all my limbs, so you don't know what to do with me." There may have been some truth in my tantrum. "If I was missing one, you would know how to take care of me, but I have got my arms and legs, so you don't know what to do with me." It is true that most of those in therapy were missing at least one limb.

One thing which particularly irritated me was the weekly ritual at St. Francis. It wasn't actually a ritual, but in the minds of many patients, it was! Each week all of us in therapy would be paraded before the residents and doctors so that the medical staff could note individual progress. My hospital buddy, Dan, called it the Parade of the Morons. From a rehabilitation standpoint, the parade of the morons was necessary, but to many of us patients it, like much of any hospital routine, was just plain demoralizing.

One week in the parade, I had a neck collar because I couldn't even hold my head up. The next week it would be gone. That would be considered progress, but in the same parade I would be minus the neck collar and sporting a new arm brace. Then the "big day" arrived, if you could call it that, the day when I had braces made for my legs. I had been wearing leg braces for awhile, but they were the generic, one size fits all, kind. They were very awkward and very hard to walk with.

After wearing the hospital's beat-up Volkswagon braces, my new custom made one's were like a brand new Cadillac with all the wonderful beautiful accessories. They must have cost around $5,000 then, so you can imagine how expensive they would be in today's inflationary world. Had it not been for Frank's insurance, we would still be paying off those braces today!

After spending my life bouncing between a bed and a wheelchair, my new custom-made braces, along with a walker, gave me new freedom and independence. Soon, I was also taught how to use my new forearm crutches. It was all part of my therapy and rehabilitation working up to graduation day. And that day did eventually arrive. It was just like high school graduation all over again, a really big deal in my life, because I knew I would finally be able to walk away from it and go home.

With the new mobility provided by the leg braces, the walker and forearm crutches, my world began to grow again. I could now get around without having to depend on somebody else. I could hardly wait for Frank to come and visit. This day above all days I was somewhat happy. I was going to be able to go home. A cripple yes, but I was going home.

When he came through the door I yelled, "Frank honey, I will be able to go home in about a week. Can you believe it? In just one week I will be home with you."

"Yes, honey, that will be wonderful," was his reply. He stood there smiling and looked at all the contraptions that were on my body. What a mess for a wife. I was down to 89 pounds, leg braces to my crotch, forearm crutches and could only stand and walk like a tin soldier. How he ever survived, I will to this day never know. Only God holds that secret.

Graduation Day arrived and each of us who graduated shared the other's pride of accomplishment. It hurt me that my buddy Danny was never able to walk. He was paralyzed from the waist down and remained confined to a wheel chair. Danny was so happy of my new mobility, but I, at the same time, was so hurt that he would never have that freedom. Danny was discharged about a week before me. After my buddy was gone, I couldn't wait to get out of St. Francis and back to a "normal" life and freedom.

Danny and I were thrown into an undesirable situation together. It is only natural that we would emotionally lean on each other and share a common bond that was ours alone. One who has never been in such a situation could never be expected to understand. Frank was faithful to visit me, but how it must have hurt him, and how he must have resented it, to spend much of his time alone with me hearing that "Danny did this and Danny did that, and Danny and I did so and so."

On the day that Frank took me home from St. Francis, as we left the hospital, I burst into tears. "Why are you crying?" Frank asked. "Is it because your boyfriend isn't going home with you?" That was the only time that I ever got a hint of the emotional strain Frank had been under, too.

It was decided that I would stay with Mom and Dad until I regained some of my strength. It would be foolish to think that I could just plop back into the wife-mother role after such a long time away. I was totally exhausted after the 80 mile ride back home from St. Francis in Pittsburgh. I then reluctantly conceded it was best for me to stay with my parents for a while, maybe for a few days.

In a week or so, I returned home. But instead of Mom taking care of me at her house, she was now taking care of me at our house. She had to come over and clean my house, fix the meals, and Dad would come over after work for supper.

It was still winter and quite cold. Frank and I were going out more, shopping and just driving around. It was so good to be breathing the air of freedom once again. When we got to the shopping mall, the parking lot was so large that Frank said, "Honey, I have put the wheel chair in the truck for you. You know that you can't walk to the stores." I realized that there was no way that I could walk, he was right. I would have been exhausted before ever reaching the first store.

I looked at Frank and I could hardly hold back the tears. I really felt sorry for him. I slowly turned to him and said, "Frank, if you are embarrassed, we can go back home. We don't have to go to the mall and you push me around in a wheel chair." In his usual matter of fact way, Frank simply said, "I don't know about you Patti, but when I took my wedding vows, and I said 'for better, for worse, in sickness and in health,' I meant exactly what I said." At that point, I realized in a new and deeper way how God had answered my teenage prayer for a husband. Frank was a very special man. A real gift from God.

It may not have been until I was back home again that my deep bitterness toward God or the church really began to surface. It is easy to be a Christian and have all kinds of faith, when you are on the mountain top, ("Amen. Praise the Lord"), but when you have been a valley dweller for so long that you have forgotten what the mountain top even looked like, real bitterness and resentment can surface. And in my case it did! For those who are fortunate enough to spend their lives in a Christian Disney World, it is easy to look down on the valley dwellers and talk about having more faith. But when your lot in life seems to be spiritually and emotionally dwelling in a tar paper shack along the side of a dry creek bed in the deepest part of the barren valley, you can begin to feel spiritually short changed!

In my mind, I could no longer be a proper wife, mother and homemaker. They deserved more. I deserved more. "God loves you, He really does." That's a catchy phrase coming out of a radio or television speaker, or from the pulpit, but those words rang pretty hollow in my ears.

The braces, walker and arm braces only provided temporary independence for me. There were times when I couldn't feed myself. At other times, I was a totally dependent child again and Dad would have to carry me into the bathroom. It is humiliating when you lose your dignity in a hospital, but it is a totally helpless feeling and one of despair, when as an adult, your father must carry you into the bathroom, of all places. Yes, my bitterness was surfacing quickly and I didn't even try to stop it. I even took all of the Bibles in the house and hid them from sight. "What's the use," I thought. "Why read words which have no meaning and power. It is all a farce."

Even in my deep bitterness, I was honoring a commitment Frank and I had made even before Brett was born, that he would be brought up according to the Word of God, and that meant among other things, attending church regularly. It is funny. Frank, in our earlier days together, was always rather lackadaisical when it came to church things, but now, here he was dragging Brett and me to church each Sunday. I went through the motions of singing the hymns, going through the Lutheran rituals and even bowing my head during the prayers, but it was nothing more than a show and a commitment to Brett, nothing more!

It was just before Memorial Day, 1979, when I discovered that I would have to return to the hospital. Dr. Smith, the one who had originally directed me to St. Francis, saw me regularly. "I can tell by your new test that you are going into exacerbation Patti," she told me. "What on earth is that?" I quizzed her. "It means all of your symptoms are flaring up again," she replied. "Oh, my God!" I thought. "Will the nightmare begin all over for me, once again?"

Dr. Smith told me about a new drug. And said she would like to administer, to me, experimentally large dosages of the drug. At this point what did I have to lose?

Within a week or so I was back in the hospital. How many times did this make? I had lost count. My sister-in-law, Brenda, drove me to the hospital. We were laughing and joking all the way there. I figured that the drug would only make me a little high or something like that. "Sure," I joked, "What can go wrong? Shoot away!"

Within fifteen minutes after I had been given the drug, everything that could go wrong, went wrong. I lost bladder control. My motor control was gone. I could no longer control any of my limbs. I could no longer feed myself, could no longer even hold my head up. I was rushed to the Intensive Care Unit. I knew I was now in real trouble. My breathing became irregular and difficult. It had been nearly six months since my last seizure, but all of a sudden they began again. All sorts of monitors were attached to me. The clots and collapsed veins returned and just as before, the doctors had to slash my arm in a frantic attempt to locate a vein which would co-operate. I.V.'s, shots, needles, monitors, respirators, they all instantly returned, along with the pain. My God, the pain I felt. How could my frail frame, weak emotions and crushed spirit be expected to take anymore? I was tired and in great pain. I just didn't want to go through it anymore. If this was what I had to look forward to for the rest of my life, I certainly didn't want the rest of my life! "I must die," I thought.

From the bottom of my tortured heart, I begged Dr. Smith to give me a shot to put me out of my misery. "Please! For God's sake, please!" I pleaded. Dr. Smith must have been tortured too, because there shouldn't have been such a violent reaction to even a mega-dose of this drug. But she remained professionally cool in spite of my flowing tears. "No Patti. When I became a doctor, I took an oath that I wouldn't do something like that, and I won't. I'm sorry, but no.!" My room was on the eighth floor of the hospital. Had I not been totally helpless, I would have struggled to the window and jumped, being content to have my pain and problems end on the pavement below.

My will to live was slipping quickly. What purpose could these years of agony, not only to myself, but to my family, possibly serve. Was God totally sadistic? Did God even exist, or was it all just a fairy tale? At that juncture in my life, I no longer cared if there was a heaven or a hell. I simply did not care about anything. All I had to cling to was my resentment and bitterness toward God, or the force, or chance, or luck, or circumstances. It no longer mattered what name was given to it, I resented it.

As days turned into weeks, I was now nothing more than a vegetable with a heartbeat. I might as well have been a carrot or a stalk of celery at that point, for I was no longer really a functioning human being. Psychiatry served no purpose. I was no longer responding to anything. When a patient loses the real will to live, medication, psychiatry, even faith seldom helps. Though I didn't know it then, the doctors and psychiatrists told Frank and my folks that there was nothing more they could do for me. They were now simply doing the basics. They were providing the mandatory services but nothing more. They were seeing to it that I got my medication and three meals a day. Beyond that there was little or nothing more they could do. The nurses turned my body regularly in an attempt to prevent bed sores. I felt the pain, but my family felt the pain of my helplessness.

On July 4, 1979, as the citizens of our nation were celebrating our independence, I, Patti Besyk, was totally dependent. On that day, however, I was released from the hospital. I was being sent home to die. There was nothing more that doctors, medicine or psychiatry could do for me and to keep me in the hospital any longer was pointless. The doctors and nurses who cared for me must have felt hurt and helpless that they had failed in seeing me restored to health. That must be the most frustrating feeling for those who take their Hippocratic oath seriously. It's doubtful that even one of those doctors, nurses, or interns ever thought they'd see me again. They expected, shortly, to read my name in the obituary column. In their profession, dying was also a part of life which they had to accept to maintain their professional sanity. But Someone had something else planned for me. He knew but none of the rest of us did.

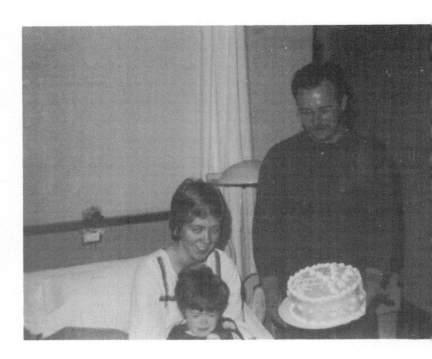

My fateful birthday

11

Patti, Go West!

Even before my release from the hospital, the professional team shared the facts with the family. I was going home, and I would die! But Frank and the folks never retrieved their helpless loved one with that fate in mind. They were bringing me home to get well. They never lost that flicker of hope. They had to maintain it. They knew that I no longer could.

Mom, more than the others, had a determination to see my health restored. She felt God had let her know that my life was yet to begin on this earth. There was an evening while I was still in the hospital, somewhat comatose and Mom was at my bedside. Though I had deep feelings of bitterness toward a real, loving and caring God, I saw something that night. Was I just babbling? Hallucinating? Was I on the edge of death and seeing the other side like those stories we've heard from people who have died temporarily?

"It's beautiful! So beautiful! It's right over that green hill, and they're singing." I whispered to Mom. "It's real light over there and I want to go be with them. Please let me go!" Mom just listened, saying nothing as her tear-filled eyes looked down at her helpless daughter. I grew silent and went to sleep. Mom related later, how she went home and shared the experience with Dad. "I really feel the Lord is going to take our girl home soon." Mom sobbed.

"You know," Dad responded, "the only complete healing on this earth is death." He was not being cruel or uncaring. Just spiritually realistic. Mom knew beyond the shadow of a doubt that my soul was saved and that I would have life in eternity. I would never be sick or in pain again. Mom also knew that it might be their own love for me, maybe it was a selfish love, which wanted to keep me on this earth. That very night Mom shared her deepest feelings and frustrations with God Almighty. She prayed a prayer of relinquishment. "Thank you, dear Lord, for giving us Patti." She thanked God for the privilege of having a daughter entrusted to them, and for the healthy years that she'd had. "I know that children are a gift from You, God, and I pray that we've raised Patti pleasing in Your sight, but if this is what Patti was talking about, and if You want to take her home, we are giving her back." Mom's conversation with God was from the deepest part of her spiritual being. "If that's what You choose to do, Lord, we won't be ecstatic, but we'll know it's Your will. We will miss our little girl, but whatever You decided is all right with us." It ripped Mom apart inside to pray such a risky prayer, but it was a prayer she had to pray.

That night Mom's faith was renewed and strengthened. She felt if I was going to die, I would have died that very night. I did not die, and Mom knew that God had heard and answered her prayer. Their daughter was coming home to get well, not die!

I returned to my more familiar surroundings, but I was not zapped with a supernatural renewal of health. In fact, I was more helpless than ever. I was staying with Mom and Dad so that they could watch me round the clock.

I was now a total invalid. Mom was shopping with

Brett. The July sun was warm and the day beautiful. Dad spent hours working with his flowers. He thought the sun would be good for me, so he carried me out to the hammock where he could watch me, and vice versa, as he lovingly attended to his flower garden.

I quickly fell asleep in the hammock. The sun was hot. Dad got involved in his flowers and forgot to turn me. I couldn't turn over on my own. The result was sad, but humorous. I ended up with a sunburn on exactly half of my body. On one side I was snow white and bright red on the other.

Mom, Dad, Frank, and Brett, once again adapted and responded to the situation in love. They didn't understand it, but accepted it. I was not their cross to bear. They never looked at me that way. Maybe the situation was a cross of sorts, but they never transferred those feelings of hurt or frustration to me. Their cross remained the situation, not me. Their simple, quiet faith displayed true Christ-like love.

Brett was now five and entering kindergarten. Dad spent most nights sleeping upright in a chair and I slept on the couch just a few feet away. I will never forget his deep love for me. This rugged coal miner was not a man of outward emotion, but he lived his love for his family. I was blessed with real love, not a brand of Christianity which is simply worn on the sleeve, but goes no deeper. Their faith was simple, but it had wheels, not just holy words. Had it not been for the love-laced faith of my small family, I may never have survived those months, for I had no faith of my own to hang on to.

"I want to go home." I announced one day. I still couldn't stand or walk or do much of anything for myself. My independent streak demanded that I be in my own home. It was total folly, but my folks and Frank once again consented, knowing it would mean double the work for all of them! For Mom, it meant spending most of her time at my house while neglecting her own. Brett was just starting kindergarten, so it also meant dressing him, taking him to the bus stop, and picking him up again just a few hours later. If Frank's shift was right, he could take Bret or pick him up, but more often than not, the burden was Mom's. She never complained, and how she managed to do it all, God only knows. I never will.

Pastor Clark was faithful in coming to visit me. His faithfulness only brought out my deepest religious resentments. When I would see his car sputtering up the road leading to our house, my first thought would be, "Oh no! Why is he coming here?" I simply did not want to hear his religious jargon and didn't want him praying for me. It was out of courtesy, not faith, which forced me to endure Pastor Clark's visits. But, God bless him, he kept coming and coming and coming.

The two of us would sit on the front porch. Locked up in my braces, I could not escape this holy man. So I sat, half listened, and was determined to endure. Before reading the Scripture, the pastor said, "I came across a Scripture and I want to read it to you." My mind was not receptive, but I always tried to be polite. Pastor Clark read from Acts, the account of the Apostles Peter and John, where they prayed for the lame man outside the gates of the temple. This beggar was asking for alms, but all Peter and John had to offer was prayer for his healing. The alms seeker immediately, according to the Bible, was healed and stood up, leaping and walking, and went into the temple praising the Lord.

"Yeah," my sour spirit rebelled, "but that was centuries ago. That never happens today." I had to force myself to continue to be polite, listening to the country preacher. But my mind was thinking, "I'll really throw him for a real curve if I tell him." You don't talk about hearing voices to a man of the cloth. At one point, while confined to St. Francis, I did hear a voice, whether real or imagined. I wondered if I was going crazy then, but now was the perfect time to spring it on Pastor Clark, if for no other reason than shock value.

"Patti, go west," was what the voice said to me. Nothing else. Simply "Patti, go west." In the history books, we are all familiar with the words, "Go west, young man, go west." Was it history and hallucination playing tricks on my brain then? Again and again, whether reading a book or lying in my hospital bed alone, I kept hearing that command. I thought it would blow Pastor Clark's mind when I said to him, "Pastor Clark, while I was at St. Francis hospital, I heard a voice say to me many times, 'Patti, go west.' Do you think that could have been God or am I crazy?"

"Patti, the Scripture tells of us receiving words of knowledge. Well, you will now have to pray for understanding to know what that voice is telling you to do. I feel that it must be the voice of the Lord." the preacher responded. Well, that was the last thing I wanted to hear. Here I thought it would blow him out of his saddle. But it didn't. Here he is coming up with this God stuff. If Pastor Clark had outright rejected me or found some demon in my voice, I could have dealt with it, but to leave me with the possibility that it may have been the voice of the Lord, no way! I didn't want any more of that religious stuff spewed on me.

The little Lutheran congregation held healing services every Wednesday morning. Though I had attended some of these, Pastor Clark extended the invitation to me again and again. In my mind, it was like a slap on the face. How dare this preacher invite me to a healing service when I had been to many over the years and my condition had reached rock bottom! My mind was saying, "Hey, the more you people pray for me, the sicker I get, so lay off!"

My numbed subconscious mind remembered special touches in some of the past services, but that was before I was diagnosed with MS and my other medical realities. My conscious mind was filled with nothing but bitterness. It was that bitterness which kept me away from the Wednesday morning healing services, or the Sunday morning worship. Where does one go from being on fire, to lukewarm, to cold spiritually? A critical observer, a genuinely holy person, might be able to diagnose the beginnings of a spiritual decline. To the person walking the desert path though, it gradually happens, and if there is a definite point, it becomes lost in the daily clawing simply to emotionally, physically or spiritually survive. God are you there? Or better yet, ARE YOU?

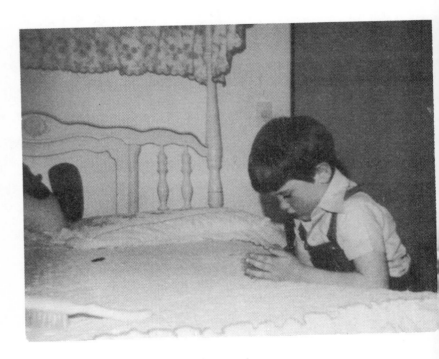

My prayer partner, Brett

12

Gone! In The Name Of Jesus

Mom never lost hope that her prayer of relinquishment had been answered when I had not died that night at the hospital. Though she may not have fully understood my bitterness toward God, she kept gently encouraging me to attend one of the Wednesday morning healing services with her, once again! Finally I consented. It was not due to any feeling of faith, but simply as an act of love for Mom who had quietly displayed real Christian love in spite of me.

"OK Mom," I finally halfheartedly agreed, "I'll go." I felt I owed her that much. That particular morning Mom came over to help me get ready. She put my shoes on without the leg braces. "I've got to have my braces on before the shoes go on." I told her. "Have you ever tried standing without the braces?" she asked. "Of course not! I have to have my braces to stand." I curtly answered. "Well, just try it once." Mom encouraged. "OK, if you're ready to catch me if I fall." Mom agreed, I tried, and we both fell, nearly knocking over the television set. My legs were like twigs by that time, no strength, no muscle tone. Nothing! They were simply useless, rubber-like growths uselessly extending from my lower torso.

The shoes and braces in place, we departed for the tiny Lutheran church. There were five steps leading up to the door. There I sat at the bottom of them in my wheelchair and braces. With all that metal, there was no such thing as the quiet entry that I had hoped for. It took about four adults to lift me and the chair to carry me up the steps and into the church.

Once inside the building, I was able to lock my brace joints in place and with the aid of cane in one hand and Mom steadying my other arm, I was able to steady myself as we slowly walked. Just as I was eyeing a spot at the rear of the church, Mom piped up with, "I want to sit up front." "Oh, great," I thought, "just what I need." So we inched our way to the front pew. I released the brace locks enabling me to fall into the pew, with a loud thud.

There was never any set order to the healing services. They would generally begin with prayer and worship, the congregation would sing a few songs of praise. Usually that was followed by a sharing period. Individuals, as they felt led, would stand and tell what God had done in their lives or tell about prayers which had been answered.

I sat there bitterly contemplating all I did not have to be thankful for. As I brooded, that voice inside me spoke again. The husky voice had never said anything other than, "Patti, go west." Now , however it said, "Patti, STAND UP!" "For what?" I silently argued. "It will take me twenty minutes to stand up and then what am I supposed to do once I am up?"

Almost instantly a woman near me stood, praising God for her son. She had had him rather late in life for child-bearing and was a severe diabetic, so the doctor had given her little chance of having a healthy baby. But the child was born completely healthy and she was now giving thanks to God. I smugly thought to myself, "See, that voice was not talking to me. I was not supposed to stand up. Somebody else did."

The woman who was giving thanks no sooner sat down than it happened again. "Patti, I SAID STAND UP!" At that point, I was literally thrust to my feet. One instant I was sitting. The next I was on my feet, literally up as if struck by a bolt of lightning. No one assisted me and had I attempted to arise on my own, it would have been a slow and painful process involving twisting around to use the back of the pew as I awkwardly tried to get up. Clank, clank, the gravity rings snapped down, locking my brace joints into place. Just as I could not have risen on my own, with the gravity rings down, I could not sit down again, though I really wanted to crawl under the pew at this point of the service.

I stood there a second, or perhaps minutes, for all I know, not knowing what to do. "All right Patti, give thanks," the mysterious voice told me. I knew that the Scriptures command Christians to "give thanks in all things." I figured if you had a cold, you could thank the Lord you did not have pneumonia, or if your car wouldn't run, you could at least thank God you had a car. But what did I Patti Besyk have to be thankful for?

The voice inside me gave me the first few words, and I stood there, my legs locked in a standing position, hearing myself say, "I want to thank the Lord for allowing me to have Multiple Sclerosis." After those first few words, I began speaking freely and on my own. "I know the Lord does not make us sick. He is a God of love, and our God does not make us sick or hurt us. But truly deep in my heart I feel that He can allow things to happen because He knows the outcome and the effect it will have in our lives."

My words began to flow like sweet honey. "Through this illness, I have realized how many blessings I have always taken for granted, never realizing..." I began to praise and thank the Lord for my wonderful husband, for at that point I realized what a truly wonderful husband Frank had been. Throughout my long illness, Frank had faithfully stood by my side. Many men would have turned tail and run away when the going got tough, but Frank stood calm and steady! It was not until that instant that I fully realized how God had answered my sincere prayer many years ago for a Christian husband. I was just a young girl in Catechism class, but I had prayed that God would give me a good Christian husband, and He did just that! He is no respecter of persons, but deeply loves the sincerity of a person's heart.

My verbal thanksgiving feast continued. I praised the Lord for Brett. The little guy always knew his mother was different from other moms. I couldn't run and play, but Brett never badgered me or cried because I couldn't be like other mothers. He was content to color or play with his little cars in the presence of his crippled mother. I also gave thanks for the family of faithful friends in the Jerome Lutheran congregation who lived their Christian love and put feet on their prayers during my illness. They were always available. Talk about available, I will never understand how my family endured. They were ever constant to help any way. I was often cruel and they still kept coming. Love is truly actions not words. My entire family proved that to me time and time again. Thanks everyone for loving me so very special!

With each praise offering to God from my lips, more and more of the bitterness left my body. Finally, I finished and wanted to sit down, a new person. My heart of stone had been replaced with a new, warm, wonderful heart, filled with true love and gratitude.

Before I could sit down, I had to reach down to pull the gravity rings up so the knee hinges of my braces would bend. When I touched the metal, I screeched, "Ouch." "What's the matter, did you get pinched on the rings?" Mom asked. "No, they burned me," I replied.

I couldn't even touch the metal. Mom reached over and unhinged them, feeling no heat. I sat down, my heart pounding, because I knew something supernatural was about to happen. When the invitation came to go to the altar for prayer, it would have taken a team of horses to keep me from responding.

The invitation came, and Mom steadied me as I walked the few steps to the altar. I reached down and again unhinged the gravity rings so that I could kneel. There was no heat this time. Since there was no actual muscle control, I rather plopped down into a kneeling position. With braces, you couldn't go from a standing to a sitting or kneeling position slowly, or gracefully. Just plop.

I knelt, a humbled person. My bitterness was gone. I was now in the presence of the Lord, and after a very long time of feeling far away from Him, my heart was again open to receive.

Pastor Clark came over to me and talked softly to me saying, "Patti, I am so glad that you came today. I sincerely believe that the Lord has something very special for you today. He has already done some marvelous things in your heart. Hasn't He?"

"Yes, Pastor Clark. All of my hate, bitterness and unbelief are gone." I replied.

Healing services in our church have always been quiet and confidential. When the pastor prayed with or for you, it was not a spectacle for an audience. It was just between you, him and the Lord. "Is there anything special for which you would like me to pray, Patti?" Pastor Clark quietly asked me. "Yes," I answered, "I want the multiple sclerosis to be gone. I want my legs back. I want all the sickness completely out of my body. All of it!"

At this point, many preachers might have used one of their holy stock lines, like, "Well, my child, if it is the Lord's will." But Pastor Clark didn't offer me any sort of a copout. "This is like music to my ears." he said encouraging me. I then boldly said to Pastor Clark, "I want everyone that is here to pray for me." It is so easy to settle for crumbs, when the Lord wants to give you the whole tray of cookies. I somehow, now, knew that and was boldly expecting His divine answer to my prayer. As I knelt, I was open to receive, my heart and spirit were open, pure and ready.

The pastor stood up from where we were kneeling and announced, "I want everyone to come up to the front. Patti has requested that we all pray for her. I want you to touch Patti, and if you can not touch her, touch the person next to you." Pastor Clark was expecting a miracle, too. "I want this to be a sweet and powerful gathering; everyone in contact with Patti."

Every person in the church moved to the altar. "Now, we are all going to pray in agreement. We all must agree on this." Hands began to touch me, and those which could not get close enough to me simply touched the person next to them. Every member of the congregation was, indirectly, touching one another. You could almost physically feel the power and presence of the Lord pulsating through the sanctuary. It was as thick as Heavenly Oil being poured over the entire body of believers.

Pastor Clark then began to pray for me, his hands on my head. Oddly enough, he did not initially pray for me, but for Frank. He prayed that God would give Frank strength in his faith, because he works in a steel mill and is in the midst of a lot of hard, tough guys. The pastor prayed that Frank would have the strength of conviction to say, "Hey, I've taken my wife to doctors and hospitals all over Pennsylvania, and I know the Lord healed her." Then he prayed for Brett, that he would accept this miracle as a small child accepts other things in their lives. Simply that Jesus did it.

After that, Pastor prayed for me. "Satan, in the name of Jesus, I bind you that in no way can you interfere with this healing. We are taking Patti under the blood of Jesus. Now, Lord Jesus, just incapsulate her completely." His prayer was not iffy or lacking spiritual backbone. "In the name of Jesus, I command the multiple sclerosis to leave her body, to leave her limbs straight and strong and whole, as they were created to be."

Then and there, I was slain in the Spirit. I slumped over the altar, remaining that way for a few minutes. Though Pastor Clark knew it was a spiritual reality, most in the Lutheran denomination have not witnessed the experience.

"Don't be afraid," Pastor comforted the congregation, "this is beautiful. Let her go as long as she doesn't hurt herself. But don't be afraid." I remained slumped over the altar a few minutes longer. I then stretched my legs straight out in front of me. My eyes opened and I began to scream, a terrified scream, "Someone, please, take the braces off my legs! They are burning me! They are burning me!"

A few of the women nearest to me knelt down and removed my shoes, then slid the braces off. The hand of the Holy Spirit lifted from me. I had had blackouts and been unconscious enough times to know this was different. I had not had a blackout, or been knocked out, or was I unconscious. It was very different. When His hand was lifted, there I sat in front of the altar with my legs stretched out in front of me, a sock here, a shoe there, and no feeling of humiliation at not being properly dressed for church.

A woman was kneeling at my feet, openly praising the Lord. It all suddenly seemed so normal. "Hallelujah! Thank you, Jesus! Glory be to God!" I looked up at Mom. Tears were streaming down my mother's cheeks. I stretched out my arms and grasped Mom's hand and stood up and walked back to the pew and sat down. This was the first time in four and a half years that I had walked without braces, crutches or a walker.

Though there was a volcano of emotions exploding inside me, I could not, at that point, speak even a word. It was all too Holy, too wonderful. I was healed, and I knew it, but at that moment I was too awe struck to speak or even groan. Pastor, in his deep yet simple faith, just whispered, "Thank you, Jesus." Then he went on with the service.

After a short while, as the service continued, Mom

leaned over and whispered, "Patti, it just dawned on me. Jerome Lutheran Church is exactly west of our house!" All this time I thought my mysterious internal voice was saying, "Patti, go west," to Arizona or somewhere with a warmer, dryer climate. The voice, the Lord, was simply telling me to go west a few miles, to my church. I walked out of Jerome Lutheran Church, leaving my braces, cane, wheelchair, bitterness, and doubt behind. I was whole! Yes, Jesus had made me, Patti Besyk, whole!

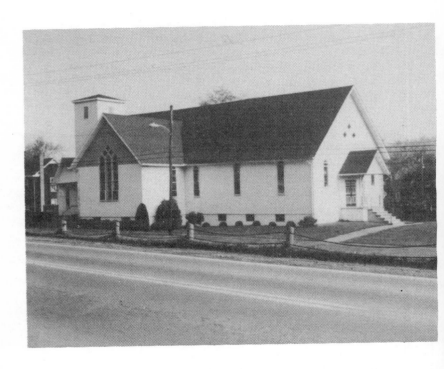

Jerome Lutheran Church where I was healed

13

Let's Show Them

My healing was the talk of the town. As a matter of fact the talk of the whole mountain area. As we left the church Mom said, "Patti, let's go show Dr. Caroff." "Terrific!" I chirped. "Yes, let's go show him." When we arrived, we found the doctor's office closed, as it always was on Wednesday. Not to be discouraged, we instead went to my grandmother, a woman of prayer. When the two of us walked in, she was overjoyed. Her prayers had been answered.

It was the same way with everyone we encountered. It seems they had all been silently, faithfully praying for this moment, seeing me walk up to greet them.

As we returned to the homestead, Dad was sitting on the porch. Mom jumped out of the Volkswagon Beetle. "Coke ... Patti ..." She could hardly speak. "What's happened now?" my Dad asked. He was now off the porch and walking down the sidewalk. When the coal miner had discovered what had happened, he wrapped his arms around me and said, "Oh Patti honey, this is wonderful!" Dad was a man of few words, and for him this was an emotion packed sermon. He was genuinely thankful to God for restoring my health.

After hugs, tears and more hugs, I suddenly wanted to go home. I cried and laughed for joy as I walked up the steps, opened the door and went into the house, all by myself! I went from room to room full of praise and thanksgiving. I was now in my own home again and praising God that I was finally truly home.

After my healing, I was not only walking, but able to drive a car for the first time in five years. Frank, Dad or Mom had always dropped Brett off at the school bus stop and picked him up again a few hours later. As I drove our car to the end of their road where the bus was to drop Brett off, my heart was filled with joy and excitement. "What will Brett say and do?", I thought.

Soon the bus arrived and my little boy jumped from the step looking for his Grandma or Dad. Instead, his eyes became like saucers as he saw me behind the wheel of the vehicle waiting for him. His little legs carried him as quickly as they could. He threw his arms around me screaming, "Oh Mommy, I'm so glad. I always prayed that Jesus would make you better." It was as simple as that. This little boy prayed a pure and simple prayer, believed that Jesus would answer, and He did. Where do adults lose that pure faith which the Lord honors? In Brett's young mind, he had asked Jesus for something. Jesus had answered, and the case was closed!

Kids are so matter of fact. That day at the school bus stop was the biggest event of his life to that point, but he didn't make any big deal of it, then. Yet, in the weeks and months which followed, this little guy used every opportunity to tell his little friends and classmates what a wonderful thing Jesus had done in giving his Mother back to him and his Dad.

Frank's reaction to my healing was somewhat of a let-down to me at the time. I wanted to be standing on my own two feet in the kitchen when he came in, doing what I hadn't been able to do in ages, just puttering around the kitchen. Well, I was as happy as a new bride when I saw him pull up. He walked in the kitchen door, looked at me, put his arms around me, and said, "Oh Hunner, I'm so glad." That was it!!

That evening Frank and I had to go to the Vet to pick up our cat. We were driving down the road, just the two of us in the car, when the vehicle suddenly began to go slower and slower. "What's the matter?", I asked. "Is there something wrong with the car?" Frank pulled the car to the side of the road, and for the first time I saw tears streaming down his face. He was crying so hard he could no longer see the road. Frank reached over, hugged me and said, "Patti, Patti, the Lord has given you back to me." It was the only time Frank ever showed any emotion during my entire illness. He kept strong and kept his emotions inside the entire time, maybe to strengthen everyone else.

The next day Frank took me over to the doctor's office. I had no medical problem, nor an appointment. I just wanted the doctor to see what the Lord had done. When we walked into the waiting room, the receptionist's eyes nearly fell out.

"Patti!", was about all the shocked receptionist could utter. "Is the doctor in? I have to see him," I asked the stunned receptionist. She escorted Frank and me into the doctor's office. He immediately grabbed me, hugging me affectionately. "What happened to you?", he wanted to know.

"The Lord healed me! Jesus healed me. I stood up, I walked, I'm fine!" I responded. "I won't be coming back here very often." I had no idea what, if any, religion the doctor professed, and I really didn't care. He had asked a question, and I gave him a straight forward answer. Jesus had healed me, whether a doctor could believe it or not! It had happened to me.

It is definitely a miracle, not a remission," the doctor said. "Remissions just don't happen in two or three minutes. They are generally gradual, and never with instantaneous restoration of muscle and muscle tone."

Miracles do happen, and I am living proof of God's healing power. From being sent home to die, to a touch

from God in a healing service, I was and am, living proof
that God does care and will intervene in our most
hopeless situations. To this day I do not undertand why
God heals some instantly and some slowly. Only God in
His infinite wisdome knows.

I went from braces and a wheel chair to walking,
running and driving a car instantly! Medical science has
no explanation. I need none, because I know Him!

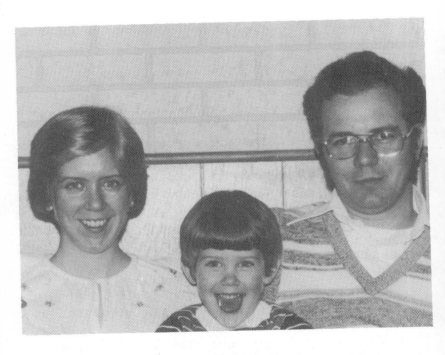

Patti, Brett and Frank

Epilogue

Through her years of medical problems, Patti kept her nurse's license valid. There were times when she wanted to say, "To heck with it. What's the use?" but Coke insisted. "Patti, it's not stupid. I'll give you the money if you want, but you keep that license up to date." Patti is thankful for her Dad's faith when she could no longer have any of her own. Had she let the nursing license expire, she would have been required to take the state board exams all over again just to get re-licensed.

In the early 80's, the bottom fell out of the steel industry, and Frank suddenly found himself without a steady job. Patti had her degree. It would have been easy for her to get a job in nursing, with a doctor's practice or at an area hospital. But, after what Patti had been through, she was not yet emotionally ready to return to that environment.

The first year, Patti went to work in a bakery. She worked as a cook, which is hilarious, in that Patti doesn't even like to cook. Along with that, she also frequently waited on customers. Actually, Patti found that she enjoyed the work, especially constantly meeting new people, and it seemed every new customer knew about Patti's remarkable story.

Eventually the fun wore off. As Patti's emotional scars healed, she yearned to put her nurse's training to practical use. One day Frank and Patti were driving by a doctor's office and, out of the clear blue, Patti said, "I want to work there." She hadn't heard of an opening there, and knew it was much more difficult to get work with a private practice than with a hospital, simply because there are far fewer positions. Still, Patti had decided that's where she wanted to work, PERIOD!

They drove home and Patti typed her resume and mailed it to the doctor. There was no response. She typed a second resume and personally delivered this one to his office. Again, no response. A few weeks later, Patti wrote a letter to the doctor and said, "If there are any openings, I want you to know, I am still interested."

Not long after that, Patti received a phone call. "This is the doctor," the voice said, "you applied for a job here. Are you still interested?" "Yes", Patti screeched into the mouthpiece. A lady who had worked for the doctor for years had just retired. Maybe it was Patti's persistence which finally brought her name to mind when the doctor had an opening. Or, maybe it was Patti taking the step, and God opening the door. Patti's miracle has touched and changed the lives of hundreds and keeps changing them almost daily. It has certainly changed Patti's life, and Frank's, and Brett's, and Coke's, and Betty's. It's also had a life-changing impact on each of Patti's brothers.

Her brother, Terry, had been raised in the church, but rebelled and drifted for awhile. He went through the long-hair, sandals, flower child stage of the '60's. He's married now. Patti's miracle touched the innermost part of his being and sparked his interest in the healing ministry. He and his wife went on to enroll in Rhema Bible College. He wanted to be a pastor, she a teacher. They graduated in May, 1985.

All of Patti's brothers can now openly share what God

has done, and is doing, in their lives. Had it not been for the reality of Patti's healing, many people in Patti's circle might have remained lifelong "Closet Christians".

Each time she sees a person she hasn't seen since her healing, the chain-reaction continues. Patti again had to return to Johnstown Memorial Hospital, the very hospital from which she was released to go home and die! It was nothing quite as serious this time. Through months of walking with braces, crutches, canes and walkers, Patti had developed cists or nodules on her hands and feet. Perhaps it was because she previously had no feeling in the arches of her feet that she really didn't notice them. But now she did. They weren't really painful, just irritating. Her return trip to the hospital again allowed Patti to be a living witness to the love, glory and power of God.

Patti was sent to the same floor that she'd been discharged from the last time. Even more profound, Patti was placed in the very same room she'd had when the doctors determined she was going to die! God had a purpose though. On that floor, Patti had some of the same nurses as before, the same ones who had to hopelessly stand by as she was sent home to die.

"Patti!", the supervisor nurse screeched, as though seeing a ghost. "The Lord healed me and I'm fine," were Patti's first words to her. The astonished nurse motioned to another nurse to join them. "You don't know this girl. You started working here after she left," the supervisor related to the second nurse. "This is Patti Besyk. On July 4th we sent her home to die." Patti had not been told until that point that she was considered hopeless when discharged from Memorial Hospital.

Prior to returning to Memorial Hospital, Patti attended healing services a few times to pray for the Lord to remove the nodules. Pastor Clark prayed, but the growths on Patti's hands and feet remained. At that point, Patti just couldn't understand how the Lord could zap her and instantly heal her of life-threatening medical problems, and yet, not remove these dumb little nodules.

Pastor Clark did prophesy over Patti, saying that the growths were very minor and that God would use doctors to deal with them. And Patti did see doctors, witnessing each time to what God had done. Perhaps God wanted the medical profession to hear this message again and again. When they hold the lives of so many in their hands daily, it is a message they need to hear, lest they begin considering themselves gods. Patti feels very strongly that prayer and medicine must work together. "God," says Patti, "gave us doctors as an extension of His healing arm. I wouldn't work for a doctor if I didn't believe that!"

A movie has been made of Patti's healing. She is now willing to speak and share the miracle of her healing and of her faith in Jesus Christ.

If you would like to contact Patti write:

**PATTI BESYK
RD 1, BOX 78
HOLLSOPPLE, PA 15935**

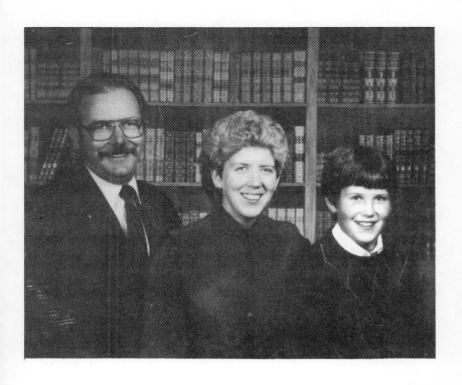

Frank, Patti and Brett